PRAISE FOR THIS BOOK

Dr Kirsten Small is the small boy in the crowd who calls out in the Hans Christian Andersen fable that the "Emperor has no clothes". She is unafraid to call out the blind trust and overuse of electronic fetal monitoring, and she does this with a forensic yet accessible examination of the scientific evidence. While "CTG monitoring is nonsense" is a bold statement to make, she then goes on to make her case and give very practical and helpful tips of when and how we can use fetal monitoring to work for women and babies and not against them. This book that will leave you reeling and but also so much wiser.

Professor Hannah Dahlen, Midwife

Finally, a guide that delivers the truth about fetal monitoring. Drawing on deep expertise as a clinician and researcher, Dr. Small uses easy-to-understand language to empower pregnant women to cut through entrenched dogma and reclaim true informed decision-making. This is essential reading for all maternity professionals committed to providing evidence-based care.

Professor Jenny Gamble, Midwife

Starting with her 'Birth Small Talk' blog, Kirsten is an international obstetric expert who successfully shares knowledge and power. By explaining research in an open and understandable way, she puts all that's known into context and into your hands as a user of medical care. Sharing information reduces fears and gives you and your health carers the ability to make right, personalised decisions that are responsive to your needs and wants. This wonderful book has been written in straightforward English for every pregnant woman, or her companions, who will face labour. It spells out everything you need to know about the choices of fetal monitoring, how they operate and their impacts – both good and bad. If they want to 'keep up', all students, midwives and obstetricians must read it too.

Professor Susan Bewley, Obstetrician

PRAISE FOR THIS BOOK

The gold standard, top shelf, blue ribbon, five star book about monitoring your baby during labour. This book will change the lives of people who haven't even been born yet. I'm equally thrilled this book has been written by the magnificent Kirsten Small and enraged it has had to be. Don't be gaslit, manipulated, or patronised. Read this book and reclaim your power over fetal monitoring.

Catherine Deveny, Birth Nerd, Bon vivant, Author

Maternity care too often relies on hearsay and cultural practice but Kirsten calls out the nonsense of modern maternity care practice around fetal monitoring and offers options to women they may not have realised they had. This book contains the information that women and their care providers require to make informed decisions about fetal monitoring during pregnancy and labour. It is easily accessible to both women and health care professionals and should be essential reading for maternity care students alike.

Dr Melanie Jackson (PhD), Midwife, Creator of The Great Birth Rebellion podcast and The Convergence of Rebellious Midwives

A practical, readable, empowering guide to making your own decisions about monitoring your baby in labour. A really important book - one to read, recommend, gift to friends - and send a copy to your local maternity service too!

Catherine Williams, maternity improvement activist & childbirth educator, UK

This book is a game-changer. Dr Kirsten Small challenges long-held assumptions with clarity and compassion, offering women the knowledge they need to make truly informed choices in labour. As her PhD supervisor, I'm proud to support this vital work.

Professor Jennifer Fenwick, Midwife

PRAISE FOR THIS BOOK

I don't think I have ever met a woman, or a fellow midwife, who's mind is not blown when they understand the extent to which fetal heart rate monitoring is so flawed, so deep is the conditioning. The reason I keep returning to Dr Small's work is because I need to keep reminding myself that the emporer has no clothes.

Claire Devaney, Doula, Midwifery student

This will be such a helpful book for women and families. Kirsten takes us through the research in such a careful way and makes it make sense. I am sure that women will find this book hugely helpful in their own decision making around labour and birth.

Professor Caroline Homer, Midwife

Published in Australia by
BTS Press
www.bst-press.com

First published in Australia 2025
Copyright © Kirsten Small 2025

National Library of Australia Cataloguing in Publication entry

A catalogue record for this
book is available from the
National Library of Australia

ISBN: 978-1-7641718-1-6 (paperback)
ISBN: 978-1-7641718-2-3 (hardcover)
ISBN: 978-1-7641718-0-9 (epub)

Book cover and illustrations by Deborah Parker, Mookoo Design
Book layout and design by Sophie White Design

Printed by Ingram Spark

Monitoring **Your Baby** in Labour

An evidence-based guide
to help you plan your birth

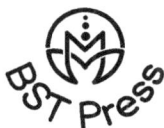

BST Press

Dr Kirsten Small, PhD

*For the women who know
what they want and are
willing to fight for it.*

Contents

Foreword

Creating space for birthing women

Dr Kirsten Small's book is the urgently needed gift of clarity and hope amidst what have become increasingly polarised debates about how to 'do' childbirth. By contrast, Kirsten helps pregnant women to recover voice, gaze, knowledge, and insight into their own bodies, needs, and connections to well-being. Kirsten's work comes in the wake of a lengthy period of the dominance of medicalised childbirth as the norm and the understandably sharp reactions to that norm.

It is worthwhile retelling briefly how and why such a norm came to be in order to fully appreciate what Kirsten seeks to accomplish for women.

The history of medicalised childbirth is lengthy; tangled up in it are stories of women's lives, fragments really, beneath the weight of unyielding institutions and the obstetric profession itself which have held the power to ignore and casually bury women's stories. This history makes working with childbirth not dissimilar to the work of archaeologists. Like archaeologists, who speak of their slow patient work of retrieval, bringing fragments back to the light of day in order to tell the complex stories of peoples long forgotten, those of us with a history of birth activism do something similar. We seek to recover through their stories, women's understandings about how important the experience of childbirth is to our lives as mothers, and therefore why birth needs to be done differently.

All of us as activists, midwives, doulas, handywomen, and obstetricians – only a few of the latter but they have been there - along with the women who have done the writing, research, campaigning, and support work for those in labour, birth, and afterwards, have seen and listened to women's accounts with utter attention. Many aspects of these stories are troubling, haunting even.

It is in the latter half of the twentieth century, that the obstetric account of childbirth turned away from birth as a life event for women, to the definition of a 'condition' that required total obstetric management. This was copper-fastened when governments came to accept wholesale the argument that all women should birth their babies in modern maternity services run along the lines that the obstetric profession had for so long promulgated: scientific, rational, protocol-based, a strictly hierarchical setting with extensive clinical and operative facilities in which they determined all needs and all outcomes for women.

For a very long time, over 250 years, obstetrics wrote its own history (Murphy-Lawless, 1998), contributing handsomely to that tradition of male patriarchy while excelling in the 'blame game' which destroyed the reputation of midwives as primary caregivers and midwifery as a skilled profession. Women's bodies were recast as incompetent by using a language centred on their presumed fragility while midwives were excoriated as incompetent and meddling.

And so by 1970, within a prevailing male-dominant patriarchal culture, governments succumbed to these obstetric arguments that for reasons of 'safety' (arguments that were never properly quantified by evidence, Wagner, 1994), all births should take place in larger maternity hospitals or specialist obstetric units. Women's stories spoke to a different set of realities about safety and care. Accepting obstetric help when needed, but not its dominance, women saw far more accurately the full range of meanings around birth. When they were given the chance to speak, they made these meanings clear, often in the wake of adverse circumstances they had endured arising from the abuse of obstetric power.

These accounts have been a testament to the strengths that women find as they give of their bodies to help their babies through that liminal space, the intricate passage from the gravid uterus until a baby comes to breathe in its mother's arms. As birth activists, we have listened to women who have experienced that intricate journey, often helped, but more frequently disrupted by obstetric science which always claims to know better and more. Thus we have also listened to the stories of women whose arms remained empty.

Women's stories reflect the zenith of obstetric power's capacity to treat birth as a condition and the hospital as a 'non-place', a 'space that people move through but have no connection with', a 'transitory, temporary space' running on its time, excluding all other registers of time and experience, with all the consequent damage (Hynan, 2024).

However, the obstetric profession has not had it all its own way. The 1970s was also the period when second-wave feminism took shape and the concept of agency and rights became central to how women perceived decision-making about our bodies. The renowned British voluntary organisation, the Association for Improvements in Maternity Services (AIMS) was set up in 1960 by Sally Willington to enable women to achieve the birth they wanted. Beverley Beech, visionary supporter of women's rights in childbirth, became chair of AIMS in 1977, and over the next four decades reinforced what became AIMS' international reputation for impeccable evidence and activism. The British author and birth activist Sheila Kitzinger published her first book of many on childbirth in 1971, revealing the ineptitude and damage of medical control over women's bodies.

The pioneering activist work in Britain was quickly picked up and replicated elsewhere, while the American lay midwife Ina May Gaskin founded the Farm Midwifery Center in Tennessee in 1971, and scrupulously compiled detailed records of over 1,700 women who gave birth in this non-medicalised environment up to 1989.

Obstetric science never apologised for the widespread damage it inflicted. Rather it slunk away, the episiotomy (it was Sheila Kitzinger who in 1981 did the first research on the damage of episiotomy for women as a routine practice) just one example amongst many abandoned practices, like enemas and shaving on entry to hospital, which were the very opposite of the progress obstetrics claimed as a hallmark of good science. Yet it continued to follow the mainstream scientific argument that 'only we can be trusted to set things right' (Bauman, 1993, p. 200). The irretrievably narrowed focus on risk, the notion obstetrics chose whereby to flag its indispensability, resulted, so far as its teachings and practice were concerned, in its absolute reliance on the calculability of the pregnant and labouring body via statistical probabilities. This was the route to achieving safety in birth, it argued.

Sixty years of birth activism say otherwise. It was women, women's voices, women's experiences speaking to the damage of untrammelled obstetric power which stated a different series of lived truths and these slowly surfaced as a policy issue about trauma in birth and birth outcomes. We owe it to courageous midwives and women scholars who transformed the vocabulary around childbirth, shifting the focus back to the entwined physical and social aspects of pregnancy, birthing, and motherhood. Mavis Kirkham (2000) gave us the midwife-mother relationship, Rosemary Mander (2001) supportive care in midwifery, Nadine Edwards (2005) birthing autonomy, for just three cogent examples, which helped return the language of birth to women.

Current birth practices within the 'non-place' of the mainstream hospital setting continue to confront midwives and junior doctors with an 'inherently unethical' situation: they 'are expected to place allegiance to hospital policy ... over respect for the wishes and needs of women', leaving them with 'rhetorical autonomy' only (Newnham & Kirkham, 2019, p. 2148). A considerable source of tension for caregivers is the extensive range of 'devices, machines and pharmaceuticals' that are now routinely embedded in the birth process (Fielder, 2024, p. 58). Their use reinforces the stereotyped risk model in obstetric thinking, while their financial cost must be met from healthcare budgets already badly overstretched, leaving even less available funding for employing midwives. As the rates of caesarean section escalate, and in many countries, the caesarean becomes the most common form of birth, 'evidence-based' care is notable for its absence rather than its applicability to the individual circumstances of each woman. Birth continues to be rendered as a purely mechanical, 'formalised' (Hynan, 2023, p. 104) process to be got through, giving rise to the confusion and deep tensions between different ways to 'do' birth and who gets to say which way.

Once more then, we need to ease out this setting, with imagination and grace. And agency.

Through these many decades of birth activism, we have created and honed the language about women's agency, about birthing autonomy, about the ethics of care in childbirth, about birth, place, and ecology. In respect of agency, we have ensured through legal activism that human rights and the structures of law, internationally and nationally apply to a woman's right to decide in relation to reproductive rights (van Leeuwen, 2009). In respect of the ecological crisis, the saturation of technologies in childbirth is simply unacceptable. Their environmental costs carry a huge 'carbon footprint' (Spil et al., 2024) which is no longer feasible in the human and more than human world we inhabit (Hynan, 2024). With pressures on valuable and increasingly scarce resources, alongside the issue of increased profit-taking for said technologies (Fielder, 2024), the obstetric system as we have endured it, has finally reached a limit.

There is an old saying in Ireland called 'on the wisp' which highlights how women in rural places in the pre-medicalised era of the twentieth century gave birth, literally on the straw gathered in from the local farm to make their labour comfortable (Farrell et al., 2012, p. 97). In her pioneering work, the artist Martina Hynan (2023) brings us to this image through a soft-flowing muslin nightdress, embedded with handmade straw, hung in the window of an abandoned cottage, urging us to imagine anew, to start again with the woman and her body in her many different places, places of connection as she births, not the procedural rigidities of the 'non-place' of the hospital. As Hynan has argued, our challenge is the 'rethinking birthplace as the merger of a co-creative process, which brings space, time, and matter into an ongoing exchange' (2023, p. 38).

While making this transition away from the current diktats which overdetermine large-scale hospital settings, some women will actively require skilled obstetric care for themselves and their babies. And so we need to think through ways of challenging the diktats and their relevance in the best care given to each and every woman.

We lost the gifted obstetrician Michel Odent only a few months ago (Warren, 2025). He was one of a handful of obstetricians throughout the twentieth century who intuitively understood the limits of obstetrics and worked to ensure that women could and did birth differently, with imagination, and utmost care (Odent, 1984). Another such was the gentle giant Frederick Leboyer whose *Birth Without Violence* published in 1974 shocked the obstetric profession for his powerful critique of their conventional, brutal handling of a baby during and after birth.

Missing in the current debates which entangle women has been the up to date compassionate voice from the perspective of obstetric knowledge, taking on board the current tranche of obstetric technologies, and surveying them critically in relation to women's needs.

Kirsten's voice, knowledge and skill, with this same goal of enabling women to birth with every care and imagination, is what this book puts before us now. Kirsten follows in the tradition of Frederick Leboyer and Michel Odent, their complete belief in women. Kirsten is not only giving us the evidence, she is trusting us to use it to the full, however each individual woman perceives her needs. When she writes:

'Anything a health professional wants to do to your body requires your permission, not the other way around'

it returns our agency to us. Her gentle, scrupulous but unwavering commitment enables women to labour from a position of strength.

Kirsten's work is part of the critical change of direction for birth that we have sought for in recent years; collaborative, collective, absorbing all the language of best midwifery practice, and adapting obstetric practice, even as Leboyer and Odent did, to create that humane alternative to the non-place of the conventional hospital.

Women's stories, women's energies have indeed proved transformative.

Jo Murphy-Lawless, Dublin, Ireland, October 2025.

REFERENCES

Bauman, Z. (1993). *Postmodern Ethics*. Oxford: Blackwell.

Edwards, N. (2005). *Birthing Autonomy: Women's Experiences of Planning Home Births*. Routledge, London.

Farrell, E., et al. (2012). *'She said she was in the family way': Pregnancy and infancy in modern Ireland*. London: London Institute of Historical Research.

Fielder, A. (2024). *Going into Labour: Childbirth in Capitalism*. London: Pluto Press.

Hynan, M. (2023). *"On the Wisp": Rethinking birthplace in Ireland for a more-than-human world*. Ph.D, Centre for Irish Studies, University of Galway.

Kirkham, M. (2000). *The Midwife-Mother Relationship*. Basingstoke, Hampshire: Palgrave Macmillan.

Kitzinger, S. (1972). *The Experience of Childbirth*. London: Gollancz.

Kitzinger, S. (1981). *Some women's experiences of episiotomy*. With Rhiannon Walters. London: National Childbirth Trust.

Leboyer, F. (1975). *Birth Without Violence*. New York: Knopf.

Mander, R. (2001). *Supportive Care and Midwifery*. Oxford: Blackwell Science.

Murphy-Lawless, J. (1998). *Reading Birth and Death: A History of Obstetric Thinking*. Bloomington and Indianapolis: Indiana University Press and Cork: Cork University Press.

Newnham, E. & Kirkham, M. (2019). *Beyond autonomy: Care ethics for midwifery and the humanization of birth*. In Nursing Ethics, 2019, Vol. 26 (7-8) 2147-2157.

Odent, M. (1984). *Birth Reborn: How childbirth can be what women want it to be – and how mothers and babies both benefit*. New York: Pantheon.

Spil, N. A., et al. (2024). *The carbon footprint of different modes of birth in the UK and the Netherlands: An exploratory study using life cycle assessment*. British Journal of Obstetrics and Gynaecology, 131, (5), 568-578.

Van Leeuwen, F. (2009). *Women's Rights Are Human Rights: The Practice of the United Nations Human Rights Committee and the Committee on Economic, Social and Cultural Rights*. Antwerp, Netherlands: Intersentia.

Wagner, M. (1994). *Pursuing the Birth Machine: the search for appropriate birth technology*. Camperdown, Australia: ACE Graphics.

Warren, P. (2025) *Michel Odent Obituary*. The Guardian, Thursday 11 September, 2025.

CHAPTER 1

Introduction

During a woman's labour, maternity professionals typically recommend some type of monitoring to detect changes in the baby's heart rate pattern because they believe this provides useful information about whether the baby is well, or not. This book is for you if you are pregnant, or hope to be, and want to know more about the different types of fetal heart rate monitoring so you can decide what, if anything, you want to use during labour. You will likely also find the book valuable if you are trying to make sense of what happened in your last birth. People who work with women during labour and birth are also going to find the information in this book useful.

When I trained as an obstetrician (a doctor who cares for women during their pregnancy, birth, and the first few weeks after birth), I was taught that certain fetal heart rate patterns meant that the baby was not getting enough oxygen and was likely to end up being harmed if labour continued for much longer. I was taught that monitoring every single heartbeat of the baby during labour was essential. Doing so was supposed to help me tell when it was in the best interests of that baby to recommend to the woman that she give birth as soon as possible. And I was taught that being able to carefully read and understand heart rate patterns was vital, because if I got it right, I would be able to save babies' lives and avoid them developing brain injury.

I started to take a closer look at the research about different types of fetal heart rate monitoring when women and their partners started asking me for proof that in their specific situation using one type of monitoring – known as CTG monitoring – actually worked to prevent death or injury for the baby. The deeper I dug, the clearer it became that most of what I had been taught about fetal heart rate monitoring was simply not true.

Here's the main point this book is going to make

– CTG monitoring is nonsense!

That's a pretty bold statement to make this early, but I want to be clear about this book's message right from the start. A lot of nonsense has been – and continues to be – said and written about the use of CTG (cardiotocograph) monitoring (also known as electronic fetal monitoring) in pregnancy and during labour. I believe it is well past the time for that to stop. You deserve better, as does every pregnant woman who chooses to have maternity professionals involved in her care.

Most maternity professionals are still being taught the same half-truths I was taught and will simply repeat these when they provide education and advice to you. Because of this, making your own decisions about fetal monitoring is currently a huge challenge.

This book was written because I want to help make that decision easier for you to make. Through the book, I'm going to provide you with information about what research says, and doesn't say, about fetal heart rate monitoring in labour. I've written the book using language that is easy to understand (and I've had people test it out to make sure I got this right). There's a glossary toward the back of the book so you can double check what the important words mean. I include insights about why maternity professionals may not make you aware that there are decisions you can make about fetal heart rate monitoring. There are tips about how to weigh up information to make decisions, and then how to communicate your decision to maternity professionals.

About me

I have worked as a specialist obstetrician and gynaecologist in Australia for over 20 years. I have worked in big, busy hospitals providing care to women with complex issues. I have also worked in tiny rural hospitals with basic resources. I have worked in private practice and in the government funded public system. I know what it is like to provide care to women giving birth because I have plenty of first-hand experience. I have also given birth to my own two babies (now both adults).

I'm an experienced educator and researcher. I have worked as a university lecturer, teaching midwives and nurses. For my PhD research I looked at a central fetal monitoring system in one maternity service. I studied the impact of the new monitoring system on how midwives and obstetricians worked together and identified what was behind people behaving in the ways they did. Completing the research required me to develop a deep understanding of all aspects of fetal heart rate monitoring in labour.

I'm now retired from clinical practice but continue to engage with new research and conversations around all things related to fetal heart rate monitoring during labour. I speak on podcasts and at conferences, and I run online courses. I have a blog called Birth Small Talk where I write a lot about fetal monitoring. I'm therefore well qualified to write this book for you.

I want to be upfront about my philosophical position in relation to birth, intervention, and technology, so you can understand the way I interpret and conduct research. I am a feminist. My feminism recognises that women and girls face barriers that put them at a disadvantage. It includes awareness that other factors such as sexuality, race, disability, and body size, also disadvantage people. Women seeking maternity care sometimes encounter unhelpful attitudes and behaviours that stem from widely held beliefs about the role of women in society.

I believe that pregnancy, labour, and birth are significant transformative events in a woman's life. The role of maternity professionals is to assist women so that this transformation is safe and positive. My philosophy considers an expanded idea of what safety is. It is more than the woman and her baby being alive at the end of labour. Women know when they feel safe and when they don't, and this includes things like psychological and emotional safety. People who provide maternity care also want to feel safe at work, knowing that the systems they work in support them to provide the best care they possibly can. Safety also includes the appropriate use of the finite resources on the planet we call home.

I am committed to making maternity care better for everyone who is involved with it. I recognise that in every pregnancy and birth there is potential for a bad outcome to happen. Sometimes interventions (like caesarean section) and the use of technology (like ultrasound) are appropriate to use. Sometimes deliberately not using intervention and technology is the appropriate decision.

I'm a big fan of using research to help tell when intervention is appropriate and when it isn't. I also acknowledge that there are other ways to know what the best option might be that don't involve or require research. For example, there's never been any research showing that using a parachute when jumping from a plane is better than not using a parachute (Smith & Pell, 2003). Nonetheless, I believe that whenever it is possible to do so, new approaches to maternity care should be introduced to practice only after researchers have done good quality research to show that these approaches really do make things better. That's *not* what happened when CTGs were introduced and the consequences of that continue to impact on women's present day experiences with maternity care.

What you are going to find inside this book

So far in this chapter I have written about why I wrote the book, who I am and where I am coming from, so by now you should have an idea about whether this book will be useful for you or not. Here is a rough outline of what you will find in the rest of the book.

Before you get to the end of this chapter, I'll explain how risk assessment in maternity care works when it comes to fetal monitoring options. Then in chapter two, I'll take you through what those options are, focussing on intermittent auscultation and CTG monitoring, how they are supposed to work, what outcomes they are meant to prevent, and how often those outcomes happen. I'll also answer the question of what research has to say about choosing to not use fetal heart rate monitoring at all.

Before I take you deep into the research about intermittent auscultation and CTG monitoring, I'm going to first explain what research is, and what makes research "good" in chapter three. This chapter will step you through how the randomised controlled trials that make up the bulk of the body of evidence about this topic were done, so that you can judge for yourself whether the information they provide is useful or not.

Once that is done, I'll tackle what the researchers found in chapter four. Here you will find information about whether CTG monitoring or intermittent auscultation did a better job at preventing poor outcomes for babies, and what differences it made to the women's births. Because of the way a woman's "risk" is used to guide what care professionals are meant to give, I also break down the research into "low" and "high" risk categories.

A commonly recommended decision-making strategy is to weigh up the positives against the negatives. In chapter five, I look at what the possible downsides of different types of fetal heart rate monitoring are. Outcomes for the baby and the woman are covered, and I also address the downsides for healthcare providers and systems.

CTG monitoring isn't just CTG monitoring. Over time, additional technologies have been built around it. These are often promoted as making your experience of using CTG monitoring better, or improving outcomes for you or your baby. I call these "the extra bits" and chapter six covers what they are, how they are meant to work, and what we do or don't know about them from research. Some of the things you'll find in this chapter are telemetry, non-invasive fetal electrocardiograph (ECG) monitoring, and computer interpretation of the CTG.

Chapter seven steps through practical advice aiming to help you make your own decisions about fetal heart rate monitoring. You'll also find my advice about how to communicate that decision. The final chapter looks to the future to see what new advances might be coming. At the very end, you will find a glossary explaining the technical terms in the book and list of the sources of information I used so you can fact check anything and everything you read here.

Some words about the words in the book

In the book I use the word woman to mean a person of the female sex, as most people who are pregnant or who have given birth use the word woman to describe themselves. These words should be read to include people who do not call themselves women but who are pregnant or have given birth, such as trans men and nonbinary people. I made this decision because I believe that using the word woman is an important part of being able to communicate the ways that women's reproductive rights are restricted. Women face specific forms of reproductive discrimination whether they are able to, or choose to, become pregnant or not. It is my position that people who are pregnant or have given birth who don't call themselves women deserve respectful care and that their preferred words for themselves and parts of their bodies should be used by those providing their care.

Scientifically speaking, the term fetus refers to the baby before birth. Many women find the word cold and clinical. There are places in the book where it is important to be precise about whether I am writing about something impacting the baby before birth rather than after birth. I use the word fetus here. Where is is clear that I'm talking about the baby after birth (or where a distinction between the two is not needed), I use baby instead.

Another word choice relates to not using the term electronic fetal monitoring or EFM. You'll often see EFM used to mean CTG monitoring. Strictly speaking EFM refers to any form of monitoring the fetus that uses electricity. Using a handheld Doppler device to listen to the fetal heart, or doing an ultrasound scan, are both forms of electronic fetal monitoring, but they aren't CTG monitoring. Because the term EFM isn't crystal clear I choose not to use it.

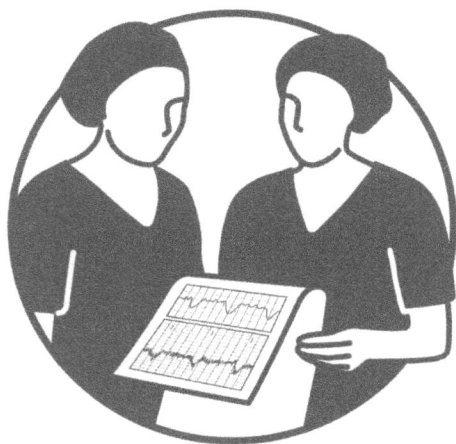

You'll see me refer to "maternity professionals" through the book. Depending on where you are in the world, the professionals who provide care to women during labour are different. In high-income countries, the professionals usually include obstetricians, general practitioners, family physicians, anaesthetists, midwives, and nurses. Anyone who has spent time and effort on developing their knowledge and skills to provide care to women during pregnancy and birth, and who is recognised by formal processes like professional registration, are included when I say maternity professional. When it is important to distinguish one profession from another, I'll name the specific profession. I acknowledge that there are other people who work with women during their pregnancies and labours, like doulas and childbirth educators. They often provide education about fetal monitoring options, but their role doesn't include conducting fetal monitoring during labour.

How risk assessment works in maternity care

In maternity care systems in high-income countries, it is usual practice for professionals to perform a "risk assessment". This involves running through a list of "risk factors" to see if an individual woman has any of the conditions listed. Women who have one or more of these factors are then labelled as "high risk". Women who don't have any are labelled as "low risk". There are risk assessments about mental health, diabetes, preterm labour, giving birth to a small baby, having a dangerous blood clot, and many, many more.

When it comes to fetal heart rate monitoring, the "risk assessment" process is designed to identify women who are considered to be at higher risk for their baby dying during labour or soon after, or experiencing a permanent injury due to low levels of oxygen in the baby's blood during labour. Here's a list of risk factors gathered from fetal monitoring guidelines from Australia and New Zealand (Royal Australian & New Zealand College of Obstetrics & Gynaecology, 2025), Canada (Liston et al., 2018), Europe (Ayres-de-Campos et al., 2015), Ireland (Health Service Executive National Women and Infants Programme, 2019), the USA (American College of Obstetrics & Gynecology, 2009; 2019), and the UK (National Institute for Health and Care Excellence, 2022).

RISK FACTORS PRESENT DURING PREGNANCY

 ✧ Abnormal CTG monitoring during pregnancy

 ✧ Abnormal umbilical artery Doppler studies

 ✧ Suspected or confirmed intrauterine growth restriction

 ✧ Low (oligohydramnios) or high (polyhydramnios) levels of amniotic fluid

 ✧ Pregnancy of 42 weeks duration or more

 ✧ Multiple pregnancy

 ✧ Breech presentation

 ✧ Heavy bleeding during pregnancy

 ✧ Membranes ruptured for 24 hours or more

 ✧ Known fetal abnormality

 ✧ Uterine scar (including from a previous caesarean section)

 ✧ Essential hypertension or pre-eclampsia

 ✧ Diabetes, where medication is indicated, or sugar levels are "poorly controlled", or with suspected fetal macrosomia (big baby)

 ✧ Other current or previous conditions with a significant risk to the fetus (e.g. cholestasis, isoimmunisation, smoking, substance abuse, significant anaemia, hyperthyroidism, renal disease, limited antenatal care)

 ✧ Previous poor outcome (e.g. stillbirth, neonatal death)

 ✧ Altered fetal movement pattern

 ✧ High body mass index (defined differently in different guidelines)

 ✧ Woman's age 35, 40 or 42 or more years (depends on the country)

 ✧ Abnormal serum screening levels associated with an increased risk of poor outcomes (e.g. low PAPP-A or PlGF)

 ✧ Abnormal placental cord insertion (velamentous or marginal), single umbilical artery, three or more loops of cord around the fetal neck

 ✧ Abnormal cerebroplacental ratio on ultrasound

RISK FACTORS THAT DEVELOP DURING LABOUR

✧ Induction of labour with prostaglandin and / or oxytocin

✧ Abnormal fetal heart rate

✧ Augmentation of labour with oxytocin

✧ Epidural or spinal anaesthesia

✧ Abnormal vaginal bleeding

✧ Fever of 38 degrees Celsius or more

✧ Intrauterine infection

✧ Meconium or blood-stained amniotic fluid

✧ Absent liquor after membrane rupture

✧ Prolonged first or second stage of labour

✧ Labour prior to 37 weeks of pregnancy

✧ More than five contractions in ten minutes

✧ Contractions lasting more than two minutes or occurring within 60 seconds of each other

✧ Difficulty in reliably determining fetal heart rate with intermittent auscultation

✧ "Any other reason that gives the maternity professional cause for concern"

As you can see the list is long! Over time, more and more factors have been added to these lists. There are some differences from place to place as to what is included, so do check with your maternity professional to see what is in use where you are. Having one or more of the factors on these risk assessment lists is common, so when it comes to fetal monitoring recommendations, *most* women are considered "high risk".

Women who are considered to be "high risk" will be advised to have CTG monitoring during their labour. Women who are considered to be "low risk" will usually be advised to have intermittent auscultation, and if they develop a new risk factor during labour will be advised to change to CTG monitoring. While I say women will be "advised" to have one or other of these options, that implies women will always be told they have a choice of fetal monitoring method. In reality, what you experience might be different.

There has been a large amount of research done over the past twenty years in many different countries showing that women are not always told that they have a choice when it comes to fetal monitoring (Annandale et al., 2022; Hindley & Thomson, 2005; Levett, Fox, et al., 2024; Levett, Sutcliffe, et al., 2024; Logan et al., 2022; Miller et al., 2022; Thompson & Miller, 2014). What often happens is that the maternity professional decides what to use and tells the woman that it is happening. *That's not okay, and it is one of the reasons I wrote this book.* You do have choices, it is your decision, and throughout this book I am going to share with you information that you will find helpful as you make your decision.

I'm not a big fan of risk management approaches in maternity care. There are huge problems with thinking that you can:

◇ easily split women up into "low risk" and "high risk" categories,

◇ that these categories tell you something meaningful about the woman's chance of something bad happening, and

◇ that offering all the women in the "low risk" category the same thing while offering all the women in the "high risk" category a different thing will achieve the best outcomes for everyone.

Real life is far too complex for these simple categories to be useful, and risk management processes are sometimes used to coerce, control, and remove people's rights. I prefer individualised processes that work with one specific person and provide advice about their unique situation, rather than approaches that lump groups of people together and recommend that all of them do the same thing.

Risk language is inescapable when it comes to conversations about fetal monitoring in labour. All the research about fetal heart rate monitoring uses the language of risk and so do professional guidelines.

When you have a conversation with a maternity professional about fetal monitoring, you are almost certainly going to encounter risk language too. So, you are going to see me using the same sort of risk language in the book, while at the same time being critical of thinking and communicating this way.

In summary...

I'm pleased you picked up my book and that you have made it to the end of chapter one. I've explained who this book is for, why this book matters and is needed, and what you will find in the rest of the book. Please join me in the next chapter and I'll take you through the details of what your options for fetal heart rate monitoring in labour are.

CHAPTER 2

What are my options?

Fetal heart rate *recording* includes any approach that counts the fetal heart rate and notes how it changes (or doesn't) over time. Sometimes people are listening to the heart sounds, and other times they are looking at a graph showing the heart rate. To go from recording to monitoring involves someone who is trained to interpret heart rate patterns using this heart rate information and making decisions about what to call the heart rate pattern. Maternity professionals then use this information to guide their decisions about what recommendations to make about a woman's care.

Broadly speaking, there are two different options for how to do fetal heart rate monitoring:

✧ Intermittent auscultation, and

✧ CTG monitoring.

There are then different ways to do intermittent auscultation, and different ways to do CTG monitoring. In this chapter, I explain the details of how intermittent auscultation and CTG monitoring are done. I'll also explain what it is that fetal heart rate monitoring is meant to do and how it is meant to do these things. And finally, I'll take you through research that has explored the question of whether using some type of fetal heart rate monitoring is better than not using fetal heart rate monitoring at all.

What is Intermittent Auscultation?

Intermittent auscultation was introduced to clinical practice in the 1820s (Pinkerton, 1969), so while it hasn't been used forever, it has been around for a very long time. Intermittent auscultation involves listening to (auscultating) the fetal heart from time to time (this is the intermittent part). While someone can hear the fetal heart by simply placing their ear on a woman's abdomen directly over the fetal heart, a device is usually used to make this task easier.

The least technological options are things like the Pinard or the De Lee that don't require electricity to work. They are basically a tube that transmits sounds to the listener's ear.

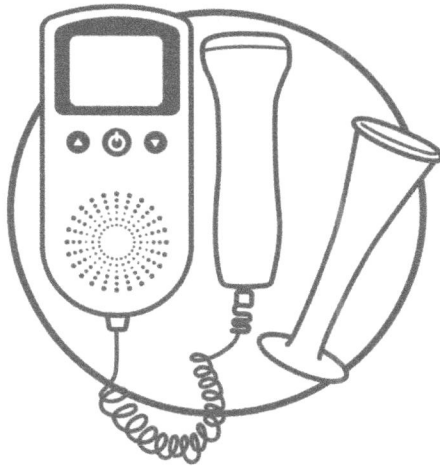

A handheld fetal Doppler and a Pinard stethoscope

To be able to hear the fetal heart sounds clearly with a Pinard, the listening device must be placed on your abdomen as close as possible to where the fetal heart is. Feeling where the baby is lying inside your uterus helps to guide where to listen. If a Pinard stethoscope is being used, one end of this is pressed against your abdomen over the fetal heart. With head-first babies this tends to be below your navel and slightly off to one side. The other end of the stethoscope is held against the ear of the person listening. Only the person listening can hear the sounds, and they are quiet, so it helps to keep background noise in the room to a minimum.

Other stethoscopes, like the De Lee, or a regular adult stethoscope, are similar in that one end is placed on your abdomen over the fetal heart. A flexible tube connects the part that is in contact with your abdomen with two earpieces that go in the ears of the listener. Only the person listening can hear the sounds. They are louder than with a Pinard, in part because the earpieces help to block out outside noises. It still is easier to hear the fetal heart sounds when the room is quiet.

Small handheld devices that use Doppler technology are more commonly used. These come in a variety of different shapes and sizes. Doppler technology bounces ultrasound waves off something that is moving and records the shift in sound that occurs due to that movement. A water-based physical connection must be made between the sensor and your body. A special ultrasound gel is generally used for this. The gel can feel cold if it hasn't been warmed above room temperature, and feels a bit sticky. It is colourless or sometimes tinted blue, doesn't have a strong smell, and easily wipes or washes off.

Most fetal Dopplers have a speaker built in so everyone in the room can hear the sound, and the volume can be adjusted. This makes it easier to hear over background noise. Some handheld Doppler devices have a digital screen and will calculate the fetal heart rate and display it on the screen so that no counting and mental maths is required to work out the heart rate per minute. There are also handheld Dopplers that generate a graph showing how the fetal heart rate changes over time, like the heart rate print out on a CTG machine.

Some, but not all hand-held Dopplers have sensors that are waterproof, so they can be safely used when you are in the shower, bath, or birth pool. If you are planning to use water during your labour and choose intermittent auscultation you will want to check that your care provider has access to a waterproof fetal Doppler. Handheld

Dopplers tend to disappear from maternity wards (they are stolen, get lost in other parts of the hospital when women are transferred, or can be accidentally tossed into the laundry), and the batteries can run flat. Sometimes there may not be a handheld Doppler available.

The external heart rate sensor from a CTG machine can also be used for intermittent auscultation. The sensor has a larger area of contact with the abdomen than a handheld Doppler does, and the heart rate can be heard through the speaker of the CTG machine. The CTG machine calculates the heart rate and displays it. If the CTG machine prints to paper, turning the printer on will generate a paper record showing the heart rate during the time someone is listening to it. For CTG machines that generate a digital display, the heart rate pattern will appear on a screen. Some maternity professionals find it reassuring to have visible proof of when they listened to the heart rate and what it was and may prefer to use the CTG machine for intermittent auscultation and generate a paper or digital record of the heart rate for this reason.

No matter which device is used to hear the heart rate, intermittent auscultation requires physical touching of your abdomen each time it is done, and sometimes you may be asked to change position so the professional can get to the right spot to be able to listen. There are then periods of time in between when no touching or repositioning is required, and you can move about freely. Note that when intermittent auscultation is used, maternity professionals monitor contractions by placing their hand on the upper part of the woman's uterus. This allows them to feel when contractions start and end, and how strong the contraction is.

Guidelines about fetal heart rate monitoring in labour generally recommend that intermittent auscultation should be done by listening to the fetal heart immediately after a contraction finishes, for at least sixty seconds, and that this should be repeated every 15 – 30 minutes. More frequent periods of listening (every five minutes or after every contraction) are advised during the second stage of labour (the pushing stage) or when there are concerns about the fetus. There's never been any research to determine what works best in terms of when, how often, and how long to listen, so all such guidelines are all based on what the guideline writers' think is best.

What is CTG monitoring?

The other option for fetal heart rate monitoring is to use a cardiotocograph or CTG machine. The term "cardiotocograph" hints at the information recorded by a CTG monitor: the fetal heart rate (that's the cardio part), and the woman's uterine contractions (that's the toco part). These are plotted to show how they both change over time (that's the graph part). The top part of the graph shows the fetal heart rate (and the woman's heart rate as well, if this is being monitored), while the bottom part shows the woman's contractions.

CTG monitors vary in size and shape. Some are mounted to a fixed position in the room – screwed to the wall or on a cabinet that is fixed in place. Some are placed onto a set of drawers on wheels, with equipment that is needed for the machine (such as straps, paper for the printer, and ultrasound gel) stored right where it is needed. You might have a bit more mobility when this is the case, as long as wherever the monitor is moved to means it can still be plugged into power. This might make it possible, for example, for you to sit on the toilet and still be connected to the monitor by wheeling it into the bathroom and plugging it into power there. Other machines are designed to be lightweight and portable, operating off a battery. These tend to be used when a woman is being transferred to another part of the hospital, such as the operating theatre, when it is considered important to continue CTG monitoring.

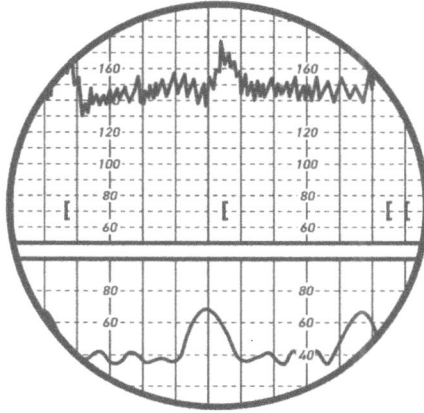

A segment from a CTG recording. The upper part of the graph displays information about the fetal heart rate. The lower part displays information about the woman's contractions.

Many CTG machines have the capacity to also record information from other sensors that can be plugged into the machine. This includes blood pressure cuffs that measure blood pressure, and a peg-like device placed on the woman's finger or toe that measures the woman's heart rate, and the level of oxygen in her blood. Most CTG machines can record the heart rate from two fetuses in a twin pregnancy at the same time. It is usual for the sound of the fetal heart to be audible when the CTG is in use, but the volume can be adjusted, or even turned off (yes, you can ask for the volume to be adjusted to suit what you prefer).

Getting information about the fetal heart rate with external sensors

There are different ways to get information about the fetal heart rate for CTG monitoring. The most common approach is to use Doppler technology. The Doppler sensor for CTG monitoring requires ultrasound gel to achieve a water-based point of contact, the same as the handheld fetal Doppler. It must be placed close to where the fetal heart is located, usually low on your abdomen to one side or other of your belly. The sensor is a flat disc, about six centimetres (two and a half inches) in diameter. It is usually held in place with a wide elastic strap wrapped around your abdomen. The lead connecting the sensor to the CTG monitor is typically about one and a half to two metres long (five to six and a half feet).

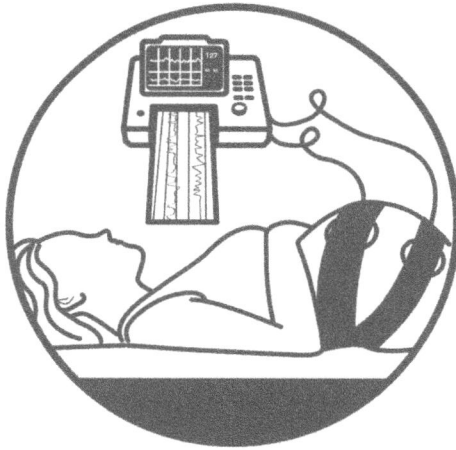

External CTG monitoring

As labour progresses and the woman's fetus rotates and descends further into her pelvis, the movement of the fetus can mean its heart is no longer under the Doppler sensor. This results in a gap in the heart rate tracing, often called "loss of contact". When you change position, this might also shift the sensor leading to loss of contact. External interference (like shower water hitting the back of the sensor) can confuse the signal. Given that the aim of CTG monitoring is to generate a continuous record of the heart rate, maternity professionals try to reduce episodes of loss of contact to a minimum. This requires repositioning of the sensors, or your body, and sometimes someone will hold the sensor in place to get the right angle, or use other bits of equipment like rolled up towels to get the sensor to stay in the right position (Fox, A. et al., 2022).

For some women, loss of contact doesn't happen very often. This means there is less need to touch you or ask you to change position than when intermittent auscultation is being used. This can be useful if you want to be able to rest or sleep, for example once an epidural has been placed. Other women (particularly those with bigger bodies) can have frequent episodes of loss of contact, leading to lots of "fiddling" to ensure the heart rate is being recorded. Some women find the straps uncomfortable and having them rearranged from time to time disruptive (Fox, D., et al., 2022).

The cords that attach the heart and contraction sensors to the CTG machine make it possible to move around off the bed. Sitting in a chair, on a birth ball, or birth stool; using a bean bag or mattress on the floor; and standing, squatting, or kneeling can all be achieved if they are done close to the machine. Going to the bathroom, walking up and down stairs, or doing circuits up and down the corridor will not be possible as the cords aren't long enough. So, while some mobility is possible, it is limited by the length of the cords.

Getting information about the fetal heart rate with internal sensors

The other approach to getting heart rate information is to use a fetal spiral electrode (or FSE, often called a scalp clip). Once in place and working well, using a fetal spiral electrode reduces the chance there will be periods of loss of contact. This means that maternity professionals are less likely to need to adjust the recording equipment or ask you to change position. It is also more likely (but not guaranteed) that the device will record your baby's heart rate rather than yours.

Fetal spiral electrodes are an "internal" heart rate sensor, in that they are passed through your vagina to attach directly to the bit of the fetus that can be felt through your cervix. This is usually the scalp, but they can also be placed on the bottom of a breech presenting baby. Two strands of insulated wire connect to a device that is strapped around your thigh. This is then connected either by a lead to the CTG machine or sometimes a wireless transmitter is used. The tip of the fetal spiral electrode is made of a thin spiral shaped wire (hence the name, spiral electrode) mounted to a small piece of plastic that protects the connection between the electrode and the wires.

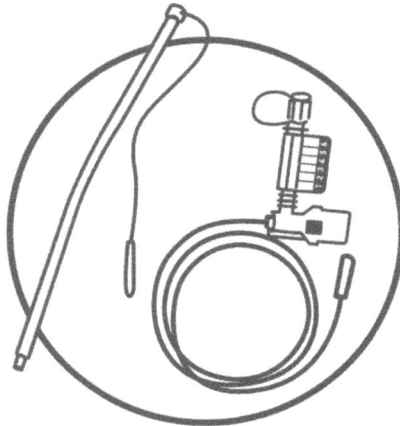

Fetal spiral electrode and an intrauterine pressure catheter

To assist with placing the fetal spiral electrode, the sensor tip and wires are mounted inside a plastic tube. The maternity professional will place their fingers in your vagina, through your open cervix, and slide the insertion equipment along their fingers into place so the tip of the electrode touches the fetal skin. The tip pierces the fetal skin and is then rotated to screw the wire through the skin surface, so it remains in place. The plastic tube is then removed, leaving the wires passing through your vagina. Sometimes the process of placing a fetal spiral electrode is quick and easy, other times it is fiddly and takes a while. If a connection isn't made or it comes off (they can accidentally be dislodged during later vaginal examinations or if the wires are pulled) then a second procedure might be advised to replace the electrode.

To place a fetal spiral electrode, the amniotic membrane or bag of waters that holds in the fluid around the fetus must be open. If the membrane hasn't already opened on its own, then this needs to be done deliberately (called artificial rupture of the membranes). This is done by scratching or pulling to make a hole in the membrane with a hooked device that is either worn on the surface of a glove or held in the hand and passed along the length of your vagina while the maternity professional places their fingers through your cervix and onto the membrane. Opening the membranes and placing a fetal spiral electrode can only be done once your cervix is open, and it gets easier to do as your cervix opens more in labour.

To safely remove the electrode, it must be unwound in the opposite direction to the one that was used to secure it through the fetal skin in the first place. If you decide that you want it removed, I *strongly recommend that you don't try to pull it off yourself – doing so could cause damage to your baby's skin*. Ask for help from your maternity professional. If they refuse, and you don't want to continue with this type of monitoring, unclip the connection to the plate on your thigh, or where the wire from this plugs into the CTG machine instead. This will stop the information from getting to the CTG machine.

These electrodes record electrical activity rather than the movement of blood through the heart. Because of this, fetal spiral electrodes make it possible to also gather additional information that has been used in an attempt to improve recognition of the fetus with low oxygen levels (known as STAN, covered later in the chapter).

There are a handful of situations where the risk of using a fetal spiral electrode is considered to be too high to make them a good choice. These include (Philips, 2007):

✧ known or suspected bleeding disorders for either the woman or her baby,

✧ the presence of infectious diseases such as HIV, hepatitis C, or active genital herpes,

✧ when the part of the fetus sitting in the woman's pelvis is not the back of the head or a buttock, or is not known,

✧ when the placenta is partially or completely covering the cervix, or its position is unknown,

✧ when the woman has heavy vaginal bleeding.

Fetal spiral electrodes should only be used for a preterm fetus when there is a strong clinical reason to do so.

Recording women's contractions with external sensors

When your uterus contracts, the pressure inside your uterus increases, and the top part of the uterus pushes forward. A tocodynamometer (often called a toco) is a flat disc, usually the same size and shape as the Doppler device recording the fetal heart rate. This is placed over the upper part of the uterus and held in place with a strap. It senses the increased pressure of your uterus pushing forwards during a contraction. While external tocos are fairly good at telling when a contraction starts and ends, they only give a rough idea about strength. Tightening the strap holding it in place can make your contractions look bigger on the graph, and loosening the strap has the opposite effect.

Recording women's contractions with internal sensors

The strength and timing of contractions can also be measured with an internal sensor, known as an intrauterine pressure catheter. Intrauterine pressure catheters are similar in some ways to fetal spiral electrodes. They can only be placed when there is an opening in the amniotic membrane and your cervix is open. A long thin plastic tube holding the sensor is passed through your vagina and cervix to place it into position, past the fetus and into the amniotic fluid. Once in place, the outside end of the tube is connected to a sensor, that in turn is connected to the CTG machine.

Compared with external monitors, internal uterine pressure monitoring provides a more accurate reading of contraction strength. This can be women with a thicker abdominal wall where the distance between her uterus and the toco sensor can mean it doesn't pick up much information. When the medication form of the hormone oxytocin is being given through an intravenous drip to strengthen contractions (you might know it by the trade names Syntocinon or Pitocin), being able to measure contractions more accurately can help maternity professionals to decide whether to adjust the dose up or down, or leave it the same.

Going wireless - telemetry

Limited mobility with a "wired" CTG system is one of the disadvantages of continuous CTG monitoring in labour. Telemetry systems have been designed to address this downside. Telemetry systems include a small transmitter in the heart rate and contraction sensors that send data wirelessly to the CTG monitoring machine. The sensors are otherwise much the same as the standard "wired" CTG systems. No longer requiring a physical connection with the CTG machine makes mobility in labour much easier to achieve. Some telemetry systems are waterproof, so you can use them in the shower, bath, or birth pool.

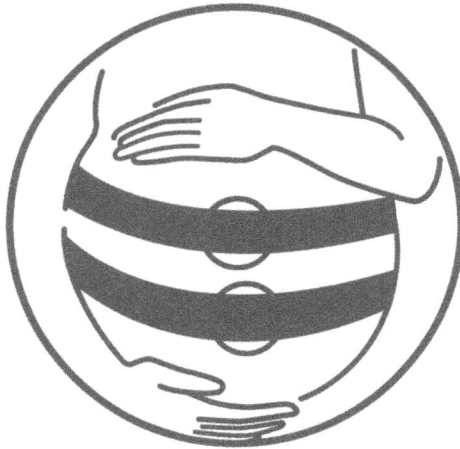

Telemetry or "wireless" CTG monitoring

The contraction and heart rate sensors run from a battery that needs to be charged from time to time. How long they can go between charges depends on the machine and the age of the battery. When the batteries run flat, you can either return to "wired" monitoring, use intermittent auscultation, or have a period of no monitoring while they recharge.

"Beltless" CTG monitoring

Devices that record the electrical activity of the fetal heart from a set of sensors stuck onto the woman's abdomen with adhesive pads have recently been introduced. This is called non-invasive fetal electrocardiograph (NI-fECG) or "beltless" CTG monitoring. These beltless systems measure contractions using an approach known as either electrohysterography or electromyography. This approach records electrical activity in the uterus, which increases and decreases as the contraction does. There's a rechargeable transmitter that clips into place in the centre of the sensors and transmits the information back to the CTG machine, so they are wireless as well as beltless.

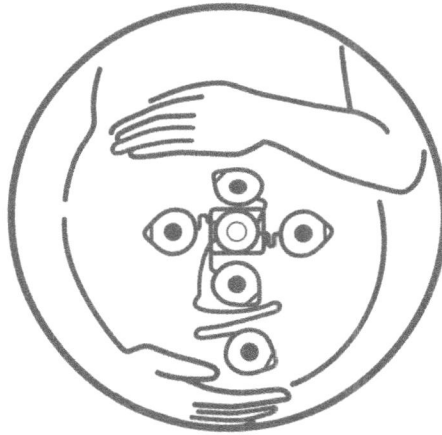

Non-invasive fetal ECG or "beltless" monitoring

"Beltless" monitors are beginning to be used in some hospitals. This option may or may not be available where you plan to give birth. They can't go underwater, so they are not suitable for use in a bath or birth pool. Because "beltless" CTG systems are not yet in widespread use, but are likely to be more common in the future, I will cover more information about "beltless" systems in the final chapter of the book that looks at future technology advances.

Mixing it up

While it is most common that external monitoring of the fetal heart is matched with external monitoring of contractions, it is possible to mix and match the sensors. For example, a fetal spiral electrode can be used with an externally worn toco.

Sometimes women will have a mix of intermittent auscultation and CTG monitoring during the course of their labour. For example, the CTG might be used for 30 minutes every 2 hours, and intermittent auscultation used during the hour and a half when the CTG isn't used. This is called intermittent CTG monitoring (not to be confused with intermittent auscultation). Sometimes women will start with intermittent auscultation and then move to continuous CTG monitoring. Or they might start with the CTG and change to intermittent auscultation, as labour continues.

Adding extra bits to the basic CTG

There are additional bits of equipment, or types of testing, that can be added to the basic version of the CTG described so far. Sometimes more than one of these extra bits will be in use at the same time. These extras are typically used to try to overcome some of the known shortcomings of CTG monitoring. I include them here as, depending on where you give birth, these may be included routinely when CTG monitoring is in use and so become part of your experience of what CTG monitoring is like. Later in the book I'll cover what research says about whether any, some, or all of these approaches are helpful or not.

Central fetal monitoring

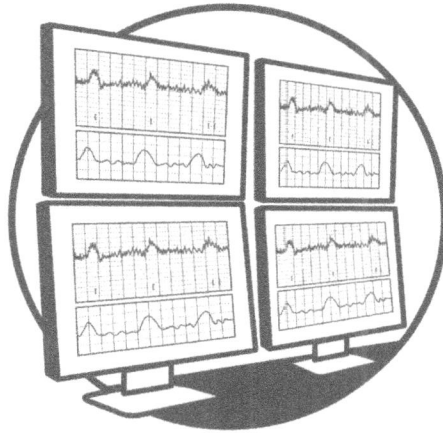

A bank of monitors at a central fetal monitoring station displaying multiple CTG recordings

CTG monitors can simply print a graph (called a trace or a recording) to paper, or they can convert the data to a digital form and display it on a screen. Central fetal monitoring systems are set up so that data from multiple CTG monitors are displayed in one central location in a maternity unit. The idea is that multiple maternity professionals will look at each woman's CTG so it is less likely that someone will miss signs that something isn't the way that it should be. Sometimes central fetal monitoring systems also permit maternity professionals to assess the live CTG feed from other sites. For example, an obstetrician might be able to review CTG traces on their phone from home or their clinic.

As the woman being monitored, if central fetal monitoring is in use you will have no way to know who is looking at your CTG recordings or when they are looking; and sometimes no one will be looking and you won't know that either. Often central fetal monitoring systems are built into a woman's electronic health record that is used to record all the information about her, her fetus, and the care given to her during labour. If central fetal monitoring is in use at the place you plan to give birth and you decide to use CTG monitoring, you may not have any control over whether your private health information is on display at the central monitoring station. Sometimes, hospital ethics committees allow approved researchers access to the CTG data, along with other anonymous information about you and your baby, to use the information to learn more about CTG monitoring (Small, 2025).

Computer interpretation of the CTG

Another technological advance made possible by recording the CTG as digital data is that computers can be trained to "read" the CTG recording and indicate whether it is normal or not (Ben M'Barek et al., 2022). This is usually done with colour codes to indicate patterns considered to be normal, abnormal, and those that fall somewhere in between. Some of these systems include an audible alarm signal to attract the attention of the maternity professional if they are busy doing something else.

ST Analysis (STAN)

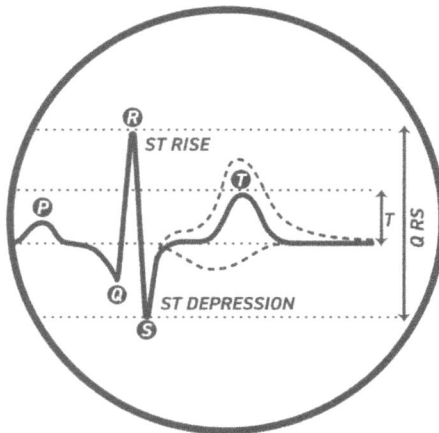

A single heart beat shown on an ECG tracing

STAN is an abbreviation of "ST analysis". When the electrical signal of the fetal heart is recorded (this is an electrocardiogram, ECG or EKG), lettered labels are given to different parts of the pattern that is produced. The S and T parts of the pattern are known to look different in adults when heart cells have low oxygen levels. It is believed the same is true for the fetus (Rosén et al., 1976). The hope here is that computer analysis of the fetal electrocardiogram can provide a better way to detect low oxygen levels in the fetus, than just looking at the pattern of the heart rate.

For STAN to be used, the electrical signal from the fetal heart must be recorded, so a fetal spiral electrode or non-invasive fetal ECG sensor must be used. Analysis of the ST segment aims to differentiate between a fetus with an abnormal heart rate pattern but enough oxygen, and a fetus with an abnormal heart rate pattern and not enough oxygen.

Fetal blood sampling

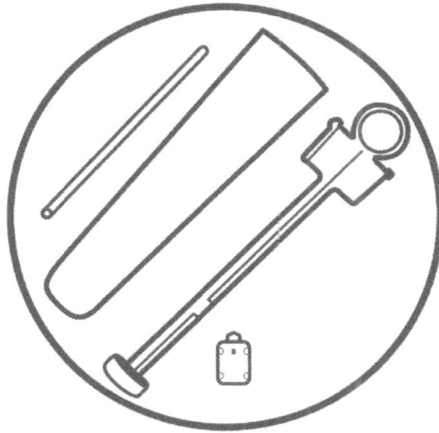

Equipment used for fetal blood sampling

Fetal blood sampling is another approach that is used when the fetal heart rate pattern is abnormal, with the aim of separating the fetus who really does have low oxygen levels from one who has enough oxygen to remain healthy during labour. In some places, fetal blood sampling is never used, or is used very rarely. In a recent Australian study, fetal blood sampling was used only once in the labours of 970 women (Kuah et al., 2023). In other places it is common, like the Netherlands, where it is used for about 15 out of 100 women (Habraken, et al., 2022).

As oxygen levels become lower, the way cells make energy to function changes. Acids, particularly one called lactate, are produced in parts of the body in larger amounts as oxygen levels fall. Measuring either the total acid level (or pH) of the blood, or the amount of lactate gives an indirect clue about the oxygen levels in the blood. There are also other things that can change the level of lactate and the pH measure for the fetus, that are not due to low oxygen. Drinking juice or being given bicarbonate through an intravenous drip can reduce lactate levels for the woman (Andriani et al., 2018; Wiberg-Itzel et al., 2018), and lactate levels in the woman's blood and the fetal blood mirror one another (Nordström et al., 2001).

To perform fetal blood sampling, the maternity professional (usually a doctor) would place a long cone shaped tube (an amnioscope) into your vagina and through your open cervix. This holds your vagina and cervix out of the way so there is a clear view of your baby's scalp. The scalp is cleaned with a swab to remove blood, amniotic fluid, or lubricant. Sometimes a spray containing alcohol is applied to the skin. This evaporates leaving the skin cold, causing the blood vessels under the surface to open to help improve blood flow. Sometimes a greasy substance is applied to help the blood to sit as one blob on the surface of the baby's skin making it easier to collect.

A long thin rod with a very sharp tip is used to puncture the scalp skin (like the devices used for finger pricks to measure blood sugar levels, but longer). This is removed and a long hollow rod called a capillary tube is used to collect a few drops of blood. Pressure is applied to the fetal skin with a swab to stop the bleeding and the amnioscope tube is then removed from your vagina.

There are two types of testing that can be done with the blood sample, measuring either pH or lactate (or sometimes both). Lactate monitors are small and portable and are usually brought into the birth room to do the test. pH monitors are bigger and may be in another part of the hospital, so the sample is generally taken to the pH monitor for testing. Results typically take about 5 to 10 minutes and are used to provide advice about whether to continue with your labour or to achieve the birth of your baby sooner by caesarean section or with the help of forceps or a vacuum.

Waiting for the test results can be an anxious time. The test provides information about your baby at the time of the test and doesn't predict the future. Because of this, the maternity professional may recommend repeating the blood sampling several times over the course of your labour.

Why monitor the fetal heart rate during labour?

Now that you know how fetal heart rate monitoring is done, it's time to consider a really important question.

Why do it at all?

Fetal heart rate monitoring during labour continues to be used because it is believed that changes in the fetal heart rate indicate that oxygen levels are low. Oxygen is in the air we breathe and is essential for the normal function of all cells in the body. Without enough oxygen, damage begins to happen. Cells start to be damaged and when there has been a lot of damage, life can no longer be sustained and death occurs.

During pregnancy, oxygen from the woman's blood crosses the placenta and enters the fetal blood. The fetus has lower levels of oxygen than a baby after birth and remains healthy at this low level. They have a different type of haemoglobin that holds oxygen more tightly and several other important differences in how they circulate blood around the body that provide protection against harm from low oxygen. However, there is a point at which oxygen levels can become dangerously low and cells begin to be damaged, and this point is different from one fetus to the next.

The brain and the heart are particularly vulnerable. With prolonged and severely low oxygen levels, brain injury can occur. If the baby survives, they can have symptoms like seizures. Hypoxic ischaemic encephalopathy (or HIE) is a term used to describe a collection of symptoms and test results seen soon after birth, that suggest injury due to either low oxygen (hypoxia) or reduced blood flow (ischaemia) happened sometime during pregnancy or birth. Some babies with hypoxic ischaemic encephalopathy make a full recovery, while others go on to develop cerebral palsy, a long-term disability. Low oxygen levels are considered to cause most fetal deaths during labour (though there are other causes like physical trauma or infection).

Making a graph showing how the fetal heart rate changes over time produces patterns that can be read. Early researchers developing fetal monitoring approaches decided some patterns were signs of a normal level of oxygen, and other patterns were signs that oxygen levels were low (Hon, 1958). At the time, obstetricians believed that responding correctly and quickly to abnormal fetal heart rate patterns would prevent poor outcomes caused by low oxygen levels (Cox, 1961). Being aware of changes in fetal heart rate patterns would mean maternity professionals knew when to do things aimed at improving oxygen levels while labour continued, or when to achieve birth as soon as possible so the baby could breathe oxygen from the air.

CTG monitoring was rapidly introduced into maternity care in the late 1960s, before researchers had assessed to see whether detecting these heart rate patterns and intervening in labour really did lead to better outcomes. Even though research now challenges this (and I'll share that with you later), the belief that close monitoring of the fetal heart rate is vital to achieve safety in maternity care continues to be the basis for using fetal heart rate monitoring today.

How often do poor outcomes occur?

I've included this section early in the book, as I think it is important for you to know that the outcomes that fetal monitoring during labour is believed to prevent are (fortunately) rare. While it is factually correct to say that any fetus or baby can die or be damaged due to low oxygen levels in labour, not being honest about how often this happens is sometimes used to manipulate woman to choose particular forms of monitoring or interventions during labour. When you know exactly what the chance of this outcome is (the risk), it puts you in a better position to make decisions that are right for you.

Finding accurate numbers to share is tricky. The numbers vary depending on the country where you are giving birth; whether you give birth at home, in a hospital, or a birth centre; what forms of care you receive; whether you have pregnancy complications or not; and many other factors like your age and whether you have been pregnant before. I can't give you numbers that specifically relate to *your* personal situation, but I can share some that give you a starting point.

I have used several sources of evidence to give you the numbers I present here. Most come from a large study done in the United Kingdom (UK) called the Birthplace study (Hollowell, et al., 2011), and a similar study done in Australia (Homer, et al., 2019). Both were big, well conducted, studies. They both included women considered to be at "low-risk" and "high-risk". Women in these studies were close to their due date, did not have a multiple pregnancy, and did not have a caesarean section before their labour started.

The Birthplace studies didn't follow babies over a long enough time period to know whether they developed cerebral palsy (it can take a few years for this to be diagnosed). I used numbers from a recent paper reviewing research from many European countries and Canada (Sadowska et al., 2020) for the information about cerebral palsy.

Here are the numbers:

✧ Some fetuses are alive at the start of labour but die before they are born. This is called stillbirth in labour (or intrapartum stillbirth) and is fortunately rare. This happened for three fetuses in every 10,000 births.

✧ Some babies die soon after birth. Death in the first week of life is called early neonatal death. Early neonatal death occurred for three babies in every 10,000 births. (For the rest of the book – I'll be using information about the early neonatal death rate. To save you having to read extra words each time I do, I'm going to call it neonatal death.)

✧ When you add the stillbirth rate to the neonatal death rate, you get a number called the perinatal death (or mortality) rate. This happened for six in every 10,000 births.

✧ Some babies develop seizures (fits - jerky movement patterns due to irritation of the brain) soon after birth. In the UK Birthplace study 13 babies in every 10,000 births experienced neonatal seizures. The Australian Birthplace study didn't include this information.

✧ In the UK Birthplace study, 18 babies in every 10,000 births had hypoxic ischaemic encephalopathy. The Australian Birthplace study didn't include this information.

✧ About 21 children in every 10,000 have cerebral palsy (Sadowska et al., 2020). Researchers estimate that somewhere between three and fifty percent of children with cerebral palsy were injured by low oxygen levels in labour, with the rest being caused by something else (Ellenberg & Nelson, 2013). I've taken a middle-of-the-road position and calculated that if 20% of cerebral palsy is due to low oxygen levels in labour, then this happens for four babies in every 10,000.

If we add all these numbers together, the rate of babies with the sorts of outcomes that fetal heart rate monitoring is meant to help is 41 in every 10,000 births. If you prefer to work in percentages, that is 0.41%. Some of the babies who are included in the numbers for seizures or hypoxic ischaemic encephalopathy later develop cerebral palsy or die, so they are counted in the numbers more than once. So, while 0.41% is a small number, it is probably still an overestimate of the chance that a woman who has a healthy fetus at the start of labour will give birth to a baby with one of these outcomes.

It is reassuring to remember 9,959 babies out of every 10,000 will not experience one of these poor outcomes. This number is useful to remember when you enter discussions about whether or not you are "high-risk". If someone tells you that because of a particular risk factor, your risk is TWICE as high as everyone else, it can be quite frightening. However, your risk would be 0.82%. You would still have better than a 99% chance that your baby will not have a poor outcome.

Does monitoring the fetal heart rate change the chance of a poor outcome happening?

In this book I focus mostly on the question of whether one type of fetal heart rate monitoring is better than another. But that skips over the first question we should be asking. *That question is whether ANY type of fetal heart rate monitoring is better than none.* It's a very logical question to ask, and you might imagine that we would have clear answers to this from research. But we don't. Let me explain some history so you understand how we got to a point where fetal heart rate monitoring was in regular use without proof that it works.

No one can prove exactly when the first person listened to a woman's belly and heard the sounds made by the fetal heart, but there are documented reports of it as early as 1818 (Goodlin, 1979). At first, listening for the fetal heart sounds was used during pregnancy to prove the woman was pregnant. Next, it started being used during labour to determine whether the fetus was alive or not. Gradually, obstetricians began describing changes they heard in the fetal heart rate patterns that seemed to happen more often when the baby later died or was unhealthy at birth. They then listened to hear if these patterns happened and took action to get the baby born sooner if they heard them.

By the middle of the 1800s, the idea that fetal heart rate monitoring in labour was an important part of providing good care had spread through Europe and beyond. Understandings about why it is important to do research, and how to carry out research that provides useful answers, were not well developed at the time. So whether fetal heart rate monitoring was helpful or harmful was never put to the test in research.

The only research that I can find that comes close to answering this was done by an obstetrician, Dr Walker, in 1959 in South Africa – a decade before CTG machines were available in hospitals. The question Walker asked was whether it was better to respond quickly with interventions to get the baby born when there were signs of "fetal distress" or to take things slow and only intervene if there were other signs that caesarean section or forceps birth were a good idea. He defined "fetal distress" as either abnormal heart rate patterns (and the specific definitions for these were different to the ones in use today) or meconium being seen in the amniotic fluid (meconium is the first bowel movement a baby makes). In total, 350 women were randomly assigned to either early intervention or late intervention.

There was, as you would expect, a difference in how many women gave birth by caesarean section or forceps in the two groups. The caesarean section rate in the early intervention group was 28%, while it was 7% in the late intervention group. Similarly, the forceps rates were 20% and 5%. But the rate of deaths (stillbirths plus neonatal deaths) was not better when intervention was done sooner. In the early intervention group 8% of babies died, while in the late intervention group 7% of babies died.

Now, this study is old, the numbers of babies in it were too small to provide strong evidence, and maternity care today looks nothing like it did in South Africa in 1959. So these results don't tell us anything about what would happen if the same study was done today. But this research does highlight that obstetricians and researchers didn't have firm evidence to back up the belief that fetal heart rate monitoring in labour definitely made things better for the baby. It might have. It might not have. No one actually knows. It is very unlikely that researchers will ever study this question as the belief that fetal heart rate monitoring works is now so strong that it would be considered unethical to do that research.

Summary

You have options when it comes to fetal heart rate monitoring. The options include not using fetal heart rate monitoring, using intermittent auscultation, using CTG monitoring, or using some mix of these at different points in your labour. There are also different options for how to do intermittent auscultation and for how to do CTG monitoring. There are different additional technologies that can be used alongside CTG monitoring. This means there are decisions to be made.

Deciding what to use, and what not to use, is easier when you have more information available. While there are many ways to go about producing information, healthcare systems prioritise information produced from research. In the next chapter, I'm going to introduce you to the sorts of research approaches that have been used to produce information about different fetal heart rate monitoring options so you can judge for yourself what the research says.

CHAPTER 3

How do we know what we know?

There are many ways to produce new information. Using scientific approaches to do research is currently the process that is considered to produce information that maternity service professionals in high-income countries can rely on when providing care. Health professionals are taught to used "evidence-based" approaches – that is to provide care that reflects what is known from good quality research. However, there is often a long lag time between when research is done and when professionals start to change their practice (Morris et al., 2011). In some situations, research findings are never put to use in clinical settings. As a user of maternity care, you can learn about the research and make use of it as you make decisions about your care options, even if your maternity professional hasn't already done that.

Before I start explaining the results from the research about fetal heart rate monitoring, it helps to have knowledge about how researchers go about designing and doing good research. Once you know what good research looks like, you can judge the quality of research about fetal heart rate monitoring in labour for yourself.

Starting with the question

The word research means something different to different people. I use it in the sense that research sets out to answer a specific question using techniques that are formally recognised in the academic world as being appropriate ways to find the answer to that question. Getting the question right is an important first starting point. These are some of the questions I'll be covering in the book:

✧ What is the better way to monitor the fetal heart rate during labour? Is it intermittent auscultation or CTG monitoring?

✧ Do some women and their babies get better outcomes with one type of fetal heart rate monitoring than other women and their babies do?

✧ What sort of harms can happen from each different type of fetal heart rate monitoring and how often do they happen?

✧ What do women say about their experiences when using different types of fetal heart rate monitoring?

I'll be taking you through results from research to answer these questions.

There isn't only one way to do research. There are many ways to do research, and new approaches are developed over time. Most research approaches are designed to provide answers to a certain type of question.

One of the most common approaches to answering questions about which fetal heart rate monitoring method is better than another has been to use a randomised controlled trial. It is also considered a good way to do research, as it reduces the chance that any differences in what happens for the babies or the women is due to something *other than the type of fetal monitoring being tested in the research*. So, let's begin by looking at how randomised controlled trials are meant to happen.

Randomised controlled trials

Randomised controlled trials are great when you are trying to decide whether something (a medicine, a test, a surgical procedure) is better than not using that thing or than using something else. In this case, I'm going to focus on the question of whether CTG monitoring in labour is better, worse, or no different to using intermittent auscultation. Once the research question has been decided, there are more questions and steps that go into designing a randomised controlled trial.

How many people and who are they?

Good randomised controlled trials decide in advance how many people they need to include in the research to be sure they can find an answer that counts. Image the thing you are interested in happens to about one in every 10,000 people. A trial with 100 people who have the new treatment and 100 who have the old treatment would be very unlikely to tell you if the new treatment made a difference to whether that thing happens or not. The chance of the thing you are looking for turning up in your 200 research participants is too small.

Because the outcomes we are interested in for fetal monitoring in labour are uncommon, researchers either need to include a lot of women in their research, or they need to find a group of women who are much more likely to develop one or more of the outcomes they are looking out for. That is why most of the research about fetal heart rate monitoring in labour has been done in groups of women considered to be at higher risk for a poor outcome.

Researchers also decide who they need to include to make their study work. To answer our question about the best approach to fetal heart rate monitoring in labour, the people we would want to include are women who can decide whether they want to take part in research, with a live baby, who are in labour. You wouldn't include women who were having a caesarean section before they went into labour, as they won't be making use of fetal heart rate monitoring. Women needed to be able to give their permission to be part of the research (in most of the studies), so researchers only included women over the age of 18 who spoke English (or the primary language of the country where the research was done). Some of the studies we will be looking at had additional rules about who to include or not include, such as women in preterm labour, or women who previously gave birth by a caesarean section, or who were pregnant with more than one baby.

Comparing what with what?

Next, researchers decide what they are comparing with what. The word "controlled" in a randomised controlled trial refers to the inclusion of a group of people who are not having the type of care being tested – the control group. In almost all the research that comes next in the book, the comparison was between intermittent auscultation and CTG monitoring. Intermittent auscultation was the existing approach and CTG monitoring was the new approach, so women in the control group were allocated to have intermittent auscultation while women in the treatment group were allocated to CTG monitoring.

Making it random

In a randomised controlled trial, once people agree to take part, they have no choice about which group they are assigned to. This allocation is done randomly. This is what makes this type of research a "randomised" controlled trial. Randomly putting people into the treatment group or the control group reduces the possibility that any differences seen between the treatment and control groups are due to some fundamental difference in who chooses each option, rather than an effect of the thing that is being tested. There are different ways to achieve randomisation, and some are better than others. Tossing a coin can be used (heads you get intermittent auscultation, tails CTG). But if the person tossing the coin gets an option they don't want, they can simply keep tossing until they DO get what they want. Better randomisation approaches make it impossible to "cheat" like this.

Getting the treatment, or not

After deciding who goes into which group, researchers then do their best to make sure all the people in the treatment group get the thing that is being studied. And as much as possible, everyone should get the same treatment done the same way. At the same time, all the people in the control group are getting either nothing, or the alternate treatment, depending on what is being tested.

In the research I'll be taking you through, women had either intermittent auscultation or CTG monitoring once labour started. The exact way each of these was done was predetermined. Some studies used internal monitoring of the fetal heart rate and the woman's contractions for the CTG monitoring, others used external monitoring. Some used a Pinard, and some used a handheld Doppler for intermittent auscultation.

Sometimes something happened and women didn't get the planned monitoring approach. There might not have been enough CTG machines on a day when there were a lot of women agreeing to be in the trial for example. It can be really helpful when the researchers tell us who had the intended form of monitoring, and who didn't, and show the results both according to what was planned to be done, and what was actually done.

Measuring what happened

Part of good research design is to decide what sort of proof you need to show whether what you are researching has, or hasn't, done the thing you wanted it to do. These are called outcome measures. It is important to get the right measures. For example, if you want to know whether a new car is faster than an old one, you need to measure speed, not how much petrol it uses.

For fetal monitoring research, outcome measures that have been assessed for the fetus / baby include:

✧ Stillbirth during labour (death of the fetus after labour starts and before birth) and early neonatal death (death during the first week of life). These two numbers can be added together to give an overall perinatal death (or mortality) rate.

✧ Apgar score results. An Apgar score is a number out of ten based on the baby's heart rate, breathing, colour, and movement, used to measure its wellbeing. Higher numbers (seven and above) are considered good, while lower numbers can be due to low oxygen levels in labour (among other things) (Bovberg et al., 2019). Apgar scores are typically calculated at one, five, and ten minutes of age.

✧ Blood tests taken from the baby's umbilical cord just after birth, which use some type of measure of acid levels (like pH or lactate). These are thought to provide clues about whether the baby had low oxygen levels not long before birth (Olofsson, 2023).

✧ Whether additional support to breathe or to normalise their heart rate (resuscitation) was used for the baby immediately after birth.

✧ Whether the baby was admitted to a neonatal unit and if so, for how long.

✧ Whether the baby showed signs or symptoms of damage to the brain due to low oxygen. This includes short-term outcomes like neonatal seizures, or hypoxic ischaemic encephalopathy (which includes seizures along with other signs of injury and high acid levels in the baby's blood).

✧ Long-term signs of brain damage like cerebral palsy or delays in meeting important developmental milestones.

Outcome measures for women have included:

✧ How the baby was born – vaginal birth, caesarean section, or instrumental birth (forceps or vacuum assisted births), with some researchers also recording the reason why the caesarean section or instrumental birth was done.

✧ What, if any, pain management approach was used, including epidurals. This was measured because people were concerned that

CTG monitoring might make labour more painful.

✧ Whether oxytocin was given as a treatment during the labour (a hormone that makes the uterus contract, used to speed up and potentially shorten the length of labour). Researchers wanted to know if using CTG monitoring slowed labour and led to oxytocin being used more often to speed things along.

Hard and soft outcomes

Some of the outcomes measured in the CTG research are what are known as "hard" outcomes. A hard outcome is where it is easy to see whether it happened or not and there can be little confusion about what the outcome was. Babies are either alive at birth or not, so this is a hard outcome. "Soft" outcomes are the result of a decision, where a different decision might have been made by a different person or on a different day, like how long to keep the baby in the neonatal unit. If the neonatal unit is full, babies will be discharged sooner than if the unit has plenty of space, rather than this decision being based purely on the health status of the baby.

Short-term and long-term outcomes

Some outcome measures are short-term outcomes that happen during the birth or soon after, like whether the baby was born by caesarean section. Other outcomes take a lot longer to determine. Babies with cerebral palsy can take years to be diagnosed and research must be extended for a longer period to gather this information. If people move away from the area, they can be impossible to find to gather follow up information. Measuring long-term outcomes takes time and requires you to include extra people at the start to account for people being "lost" from follow up. This sort of research is challenging and more expensive to do, but it is important if we want to know how babies and women are doing in the longer term.

Surrogate end points

To date, there is no test that can directly measure whether the baby's brain is being or has been injured from low oxygen levels before birth or not. However, some outcome measures offer clues about whether the baby may have been exposed to harmfully low levels of oxygen. These are called surrogate end points.

Acid levels in the umbilical cord blood just after birth are an example of a surrogate end point. Babies who have had low oxygen levels are more likely to have high blood acid levels (Johnson et al., 2021). However, not all babies who had low oxygen levels will have high acid levels. There are also reasons for a baby to have high blood levels of acid that aren't related to low oxygen levels. Some of the differences relate to whether the cord is clamped and cut early, or whether circulation between the baby and the placenta continues until physiological changes close the blood vessels in the cord. Surrogate end points provide approximate answers to our research question when it is hard (or impossible) to measure the thing we want to know about.

I'm more interested in hard outcomes than in surrogate end points or soft outcomes. If a baby has low Apgar scores, or high acid levels, or is admitted to the neonatal unit for observation, these can be a cause of anxiety. However, many (even most) babies with one of these surrogate end points are ultimately completely healthy. I'll be focussing on death, seizures, hypoxic ischaemic encephalopathy, and cerebral palsy in the book for this reason.

Systematic reviews with meta-analysis

We now reach the point where the randomised controlled trial is done. And then another group of researchers do a very similar trial to answer the same question, and another group. A collection of results is now available.

Once there is more than one randomised controlled trial, a new problem appears. If trial 1 says there was a 10% improvement, trial 2 says things were 13% worse, and trial 3 says there was no difference – how do you make sense of this? To solve this, researchers find all the trials and combine them to get the biggest possible number of research data in one place. They then use this bigger pool of information to calculate one combined answer to the research question. This is known as a systematic review with meta-analysis.

One prominent research organisation, the Cochrane Library (cochranelibrary.com), specialises in doing these and they are known as Cochrane reviews. Depending on where you are in the world, you might be able to access full versions of all the reviews in the online Cochrane Library. If you don't have full access, you will at least be able to see a summary of each review. There are reviews about a great many health related topics, including pregnancy and birth. There is a Cochrane review that has brought together all the randomised controlled trials comparing intermittent auscultation with CTG monitoring during labour in the one place (Alfirevic et al., 2017) – and I'm going to explain the results of that review in the next chapter.

The Cochrane review

The process of meta-analysis is sort of like making a research smoothie. You put different individual ingredients in, blend, and get one final result. Of course, the end result is only as good as the quality of the ingredients that went into it. So it is helpful for you to know what the ingredients were in the Cochrane review that compared CTG use in labour with intermittent auscultation.

All the randomised controlled trials included in the review were done many years ago. The earliest was in 1976, most were done in the 1980s, and the most recent was in 2006. It is important to acknowledge the world of maternity care, and indeed the world in general, looked different at the time most of the research was being done than it does now. There are many reasons why women and babies have different health outcomes now than they did at the time the research was done.

The oral contraceptive pill had only been widely available for a little more than a decade when the first studies were done (de Costa, 2020), and none of the newer contraceptive options like implants and hormonal intrauterine devices were available. Because of this, women tended to have their first baby at a younger age, and had more babies during their lifetime. The average age of women in the first randomised controlled trial was 22 years (Haverkamp et al., 1976) while in Australia in 2022 it was 31 years (Australian Institute of Health and Welfare, 2024).

Ultrasound scanning equipment began being used in clinical practice in high-income countries in the middle of the 1970s (Campbell, 2013). Both the equipment and knowledge about how to use the technology were not well developed, so it was difficult to identify babies with abnormalities or who were not healthy before labour started. This is much less likely to happen today.

Synthetic oxytocin was invented in 1955, with its use in induction of labour starting to become more common in the 1960s (Drife, 2021). In the UK in 1965, only 8% of women had their labour induced (Drife, 2021), while the average induction of labour rate was 36% in 2021 (Taylor et al., 2024). The caesarean section rate was much lower than it is now. In the large fetal monitoring trial done in Dublin, Ireland in the early 1980s the caesarean rate before labour was 3% and during labour it was 2% (MacDonald et al, 1985). By 2019, the overall caesarean rate in Ireland had risen to 32% (Amyx et al., 2023). Similar increases in both the induction and caesarean rates are reported across all high-income countries and reflect big changes in the way care has been provided.

Care of the newborn has also dramatically changed over time (Christie & Tansey, 2001). Ventilators and other devices that help to push air into baby's lungs to assist with their breathing were introduced during the 1960s. Premature and sick babies that would not have been able to survive before the 1970s began to be treated and survival rates for babies using neonatal care have consistently improved over time.

A lot of research, financial investment, and policy development has happened in maternity care during the decades since the first randomised controlled trial in 1976, all aimed at improving outcomes for women and babies. While not all the changes have been useful, there has been a reduction in rates of death during pregnancy and soon after birth. For example, in Europe stillbirth rates during pregnancy and labour fell from 14 per 1,000 births in the 1960s to 6 per 1,000 births in the 1980s, and infant deaths in the first week after birth fell from 14 per 1000 births to 2 per 1,000 births over the same period (Kalter, 1991). The pace of change has been stagnant in more recent decades. The most recent Australian figures (for births in 2023) report a rate of stillbirth in pregnancy and labour of 9 per 1,000 births and neonatal deaths a rate of 2 per 1,000 births (Australian Institute of Health and Welfare, 2025); in the UK in 2022 the stillbirth rate was 3 per 1,000 births and the neonatal death rate was 2 per 1,000 births (Gallimore et al., 2024); and in the USA in 2021 the stillbirth rate was 3 per 1,000 births and the neonatal death rate was also 3 per 1,000 births (Valenzuela et al, 2023).

Many changes more broadly in society have also made pregnancy and birth safer. Women are less likely to lose their employment when they become pregnant. Women can hold bank accounts and own property in their own name. While intimate partner abuse continues to be a significant problem, much has been done to address it over the period we are looking at. These and other social and healthcare improvements impact on the number of women and babies experiencing poor outcomes, and on the way that complications during labour are recognised and managed.

It could be that increasing use of CTG monitoring had a part to play in the improvements in mortality rates. Or, it could be that all the other changes were what made the difference and CTG monitoring had no impact at all, or even had a harmful impact that was offset by other improvements. One of the challenges of taking evidence from the research about CTG monitoring and using it in practice is knowing that the outcomes could be different if the research were done again today. This is a problem with all scientific knowledge, not just with research about CTG monitoring.

The studies in the review

The current version of the Cochrane review about fetal heart rate monitoring during labour was published in 2017. The authors, Alfirevic, Devane, Gyte, and Cuthbert, found thirteen randomised controlled trials. One trial compared continuous use of CTG monitoring with intermittent CTG monitoring (switching back to intermittent auscultation in between periods of CTG monitoring). Eleven trials compared continuous CTG use with intermittent auscultation. The remaining trial compared months when the hospital locked most of the CTG machines away with months when all their CTG machines were used.

The first randomised controlled trial included only women considered to be at high risk (Haverkamp, et al., 1976). The researchers used a unique approach that has not been done again since. All the women who agreed to be in the trial had a fetal spiral electrode and internal contraction monitoring. Those who were randomly selected for intermittent auscultation had the CTG monitor placed outside the room and covered so a CTG recording was generated but was not looked at during labour. The fetal heart was listened to every 15 minutes in the first stage of labour and every 5 minutes in the second stage, but they didn't describe what equipment was used for this. Women randomised to CTG monitoring had the monitor in the room and information from the monitor could be used when making decisions about care. This approach helped reduce any differences in outcomes that might have been due to the internal monitoring equipment, rather than from using the information generated by the CTG machine.

This first study used only internal CTG monitoring, others used only external CTG monitoring (an unpublished study done in Pakistan in

1989), and most included both options (for example Wood et al, 1991; MacDonald et al, 1985). Intermittent auscultation was typically done every 15 to 30 minutes during labour, and every 5 minutes or after every contraction in the pushing (second) stage of labour. Some studies used Pinard stethoscopes (for example MacDonald et al, 1985), others used a handheld Doppler (for example Vintzileos et al., 1993), some used either option for intermittent auscultation (for example Kelso et al., 1978).

Who was included in the individual studies varied. Two trials attempted to include only women who were considered to have a low risk for poor outcomes for the fetus and baby (Kelso, et al., 1978; Wood et al., 1981). Some included only women considered to be at high risk for a wide range of reasons (for example Renou, et al 1976; Haverkamp, et al, 1979; MacDonald, et al., 1985). Some of the risk factors that were used to decide who was eligible for the trials included preterm labour, multiple pregnancy, diabetes, high blood pressure, meconium staining of the amniotic fluid, hearing an abnormal heart rate on intermittent auscultation, and the use of oxytocin during labour. Having any one of these made a woman eligible for the trial, and the outcomes for them and their babies were not reported separately according to the reason they were considered to be at higher risk.

Three studies included women with only one particular risk factor. These were:

✧ Preterm labour between 26 and 32 weeks (Luthy, et al., 1987)

✧ Meconium-stained liquor (the Pakistan 1989 study that has never been published)

✧ One previous caesarean section (Madaan & Trivedi, 2006).

The size of the studies varied a lot. The smallest included only 100 women (Madaan & Trivedi, 2006). Only three had over 1,000 women:

✧ The Dublin based trial in Ireland by MacDonald et al. (1985) had 12,964 women

◇ The Dallas based trial in North America where some CTG monitors were locked away every second month (Leveno, et al., 1986) had 34,995 women

◇ The Athens based trial in Greece by Vintzileos et al. (1993) had 1,428 women.

Only two trials looked at long term outcomes. These were the Dublin trial (longer term data were published by Grant et al. in 1989) and the preterm labour trial (their follow up findings were published by Shy et al. in 1990).

In all these trials the people providing care during labour and the women giving birth knew which type of monitoring was being used. They made decisions about what care to provide based on the results of the monitoring. This means the trial was not "blinded" and there was a risk that people made different decisions because they knew what sort of monitoring was used. These decisions, rather than the type of monitoring, might have produced the results seen in the trial. In some trials, professionals looking after the babies after birth were not told which type of monitoring was used to try to reduce this type of bias.

None of the trial authors provided information about when the umbilical cord was clamped after birth. There is increasing evidence that clamping the cord as soon as possible after birth is associated with worse outcomes for the baby, particularly if they are premature (Rabe et al., 2019). Differences in the time taken to clamp the cord might have had an impact on some of the outcomes seen in the trials in the Cochrane review, but there is no way to determine what that impact might have been.

Summary

Many people, including myself, like to use information from good quality research when making decisions about their health care options. This chapter has explored some of the ways that researchers design research that is considered to be good quality. The "ingredients" in the Cochrane review have been listed, and you can probably see that much of this research is past its "use by date" – to push the food analogy a bit further. That doesn't mean that we should simply throw it out, but it does mean that we should think hard about how best to use the information from the research in the present day and in places and birth settings different to the ones where the research was done.

By now you are probably very curious about what the results of the research studies showed. The answers are waiting in the next chapter!

CHAPTER 4

Here is what the research says

I have introduced the individual research studies that went into the Cochrane review (Alfirevic et al., 2017). This chapter takes you through the results that the Cochrane review team found when they combined all the studies. Given that fetal monitoring is supposed to improve outcomes for the baby, I'll start there. Then, because it is important that women don't end up worse off from the use of fetal monitoring, I'll go through outcomes for women. I'll also look at types of research that are not randomised controlled trials but have also compared CTG use with intermittent auscultation. And because CTG monitoring is sometimes used during pregnancy (antenatal CTG monitoring) or when a woman first comes to hospital in labour (admission CTG monitoring) I include short summaries of what research says about these two options as well.

Outcomes for babies

Deaths

In total, eleven studies, conducted between 1976 and 1993, with 33,513 births, provided data about death of the baby during labour or the first week of life (Alfirevic et al., 2017). For women randomly allocated to CTG monitoring in labour, the death rate for their babies was 30 per 10,000 births. For women randomly allocated to intermittent auscultation, the perinatal mortality rate was 34 per 10,000 births. While there was a small difference in the numbers, statistical testing shows that this difference was not big enough to say that there really was a difference between the two groups. This is known as statistical significance, and in this instance the difference was not statistically significant.

The Cochrane review doesn't provide information about stillbirth separately from early neonatal death, just the combination of the two together. I have gone back to the original research and pulled that data out and analysed it. Ten of the eleven trials, with 33,313 women, provided data for this analysis. One unpublished trial is included in the Cochrane review (where it is referred to as Pakistan 1989). Because it has never been published I couldn't access it to see if they counted stillbirths and neonatal death separately to include this in my calculations.

Stillbirth in labour occurred for 2 per 10,000 births in the CTG monitoring group and 4 per 10,000 births in the intermittent auscultation group. The difference was not statistically significant. For death in the first week of life the numbers are 23 per 10,000 births for the CTG monitoring group and 26 per 10,000 births for the intermittent auscultation group. Again, the difference was not statistically significant.

Both the rate of stillbirth during labour and deaths in the first week of life were the same in the intermittent auscultation group as the CTG monitoring group.

Neonatal seizures

Nine studies spanning the period 1976 to 1993, with 32,386 babies included, provide information about neonatal seizures (Alfirevic et al., 2017). Here, the difference *was* statistically significant. In the CTG monitoring group 15 babies in 10,000 had neonatal seizures and for the intermittent auscultation group it was higher at 30 babies in 10,000. The seizure rate was half the rate for babies in the CTG monitoring group than it was for those in the intermittent auscultation group. Another useful way to think about these numbers is to calculate how many women would need to be monitored by CTG to prevent one baby from experiencing seizures. This is called the number needed to treat, and it was 667.

> In this research, women in the CTG monitoring group had less chance of their baby having seizures after birth. For every 667 women who had CTG monitoring rather than intermittent auscultation, one baby would not experience seizures.

There's more to the story about neonatal seizures – but hold on for a moment and I'll give you the rest of the outcomes for babies first. And then I'll bring you back for a more detailed discussion about neonatal seizures.

Cerebral palsy

Only two trials, with 13,252 babies included, provided long term follow up data about cerebral palsy (Alfirevic et al., 2017). Cerebral palsy affected 42 babies for every 10,000 in the CTG monitoring group, and 26 for every 10,000 in the intermittent auscultation group. While the rate was higher for babies whose mothers were in the CTG monitoring group, the difference was not statistically significant.

> Overall, the cerebral palsy rate was the same in the intermittent auscultation group as the CTG monitoring group.

Other outcomes for the baby

No statistically significant differences between babies in the CTG monitoring group and the intermittent auscultation group were found for:

1. High levels of acid in umbilical cord blood after birth

2. Hypoxic ischaemic encephalopathy

3. Low Apgar scores

4. Admission to the neonatal intensive care unit

5. How long babies stayed in the intensive care unit if they were admitted

What about women considered to be at higher risk?

As I explained in the first chapter, the current approach in maternity care is to split women up into "low risk" and "high risk". Women in the "low risk" group usually get intermittent auscultation for their labour, while women in the "high risk" group get CTG monitoring. So let's go back and take a second look at the outcomes for babies and separate them into "low" and "high" risk categories. The authors of the Cochrane review did this, and also included a category called "unknown and mixed risk". The trials in this category either had a mix of women from both "low" and "high risk" categories, or the authors of the original research didn't say anything about whether women in their study were "low" or "high risk".

Let's start with the "low risk" group. There were three studies that provide information here, with information about deaths from 16,049 births, and 25,175 births for neonatal seizures (Alfirevic et al., 2017). None of these studies looked at cerebral palsy as an outcome. No babies died from stillbirth during labour for this group of women. There was no statistically significant difference in the rate of deaths in the first week of life. There was a significant difference in neonatal seizures, which happened for 6 in every 10,000 babies in the CTG monitored group and 18 in every 10,000 babies in the intermittent auscultation group. Here, 840 women would need to have CTG monitoring to prevent one baby from having neonatal seizures.

Next, let's look at the "unknown and mixed risk" group. There were three studies providing information about death, with 15,490 births (Alfirevic et al., 2017). There were no statistically significant differences in either the rate of stillbirth or death in the first week of life, or in the overall perinatal mortality rate when you add the two together. There were two trials with 2,406 births that provided information about neonatal seizures, and there was no statistically significant difference between being in the CTG group or the intermittent auscultation group. One trial, with 13,079 births looked at cerebral palsy in this group, and found no statistically significant difference in how often this happened between the two groups.

Finally, here are the results for the "high risk" group. Five studies provide information here (Alfirevic et al., 2017). There was no statistically significant difference in stillbirth, death in the first week of life, perinatal mortality, or neonatal seizures. Cerebral palsy rates were significantly higher in the group allocated to CTG monitoring than they were for the group allocated to intermittent auscultation. This was a very small study of babies born prematurely, with only 173 babies followed until they were old enough to be diagnosed, so this result should be considered cautiously. Cerebral palsy is more common in premature babies, and was diagnosed for 16 of 82 babies who had CTG monitoring (this is equivalent to 1,951 in 10,000 babies) and in 7 of the 91 babies (equivalent to 769 in 10,000 babies) who had intermittent auscultation. Cerebral palsy was two-and-a-half times higher in the CTG monitoring group than in the intermittent auscultation group. Another way of looking at this is to say that for every nine babies with CTG monitoring, there was one extra baby with cerebral palsy than there would have been if intermittent auscultation had been used.

At first glance this looks astonishing.

The group of women who are typically told that intermittent auscultation is their best option because they are "low risk" were the group whose babies had the better outcomes with CTG use. And the "high risk" group of women who are typically told that CTG monitoring is really important for them, had worse outcomes with CTG use for their babies.

As I said back in the first chapter, there are some serious problems with the very idea of "risk" and these problems played out in the research. And that should make everyone very cautious about how they choose to use this information when making decisions.

Here's why I'm really cautious about what the "risk" breakdown actually means for babies

First, the list of things that was used to decide who was "high risk" or not was different from one study to the next, and it is different now to the time when the studies were done. There are many ways that this turns up in these studies, but let me give you just one example, using the trial from Sheffield, UK, published by Kelso and colleagues in 1978. This trial was meant to be, and is described in both their paper and in the Cochrane review as having a "low risk" group of women.

However, when you read the details in the paper, 26% of the women had their labour induced with oxytocin and another 24% had their labour sped up with oxytocin. Given through an intravenous drip, the hormone oxytocin increases the strength of a woman's contractions, makes them last longer, and happen more often. This reduces the time in between contractions when the woman's uterus is at rest. The movement of oxygen across the placenta is reduced during contractions. Because of this, oxytocin is considered to increase the possibility that the fetus might experience low oxygen levels during labour, and must be used carefully (Oláh & Steer, 2015).

This was known at the time the study was being done in Sheffield. The first of the studies, published by Haverkamp and colleagues in 1976, had recognised the dangers of oxytocin use. They included it on their list of risk factors that made women eligible to be included in their trial of only "high risk" women. Oxytocin use is also on the list of risk factors for which CTG monitoring is recommended in current guidelines written by major obstetric organisations around the world (see the list in Chapter One).

In this so-called "low risk" trial, at least half the women were not "low risk". So that makes me very cautious about saying that these results are relevant to a woman who is considered "low risk" today.

The second reason I recommend caution here is that the researchers who were doing these studies were not particularly good at selecting a group of women who were more, or less, likely to end up with a bad outcome for their babies. Risk assessment processes, both then and now, are not a very accurate tool. I've put together a table to show what I mean here. Each of the studies in the Cochrane review are in the table, with their location and the year they were published, and the overall perinatal mortality rate for all the babies born in that trial. I have listed them in order, with the lowest perinatal mortality rate at the bottom, and the highest perinatal mortality rate at the top. The colour coded boxes show whether the individual trials were described as having been done with a group of women considered "low risk" (white), mixed or unknown risk (grey), or "high risk" (black).

Trial	Perinatal mortality rate per 10,000 births
Seattle, Luthy et al., 1987	1,423
Pakistan, unpublished, 1989	450
Dallas. Leveno et al., 1986	80
Athens, Vintzileos et al., 1993	77
Melbourne, Renou et al., 1976	57
Copenhagen, Neldam et al., 1985	52
Denver, Haverkamp et al., 1979	28
Dublin, MacDonald et al., 1985	22
Denver, Haverkamp et al., 1976	20
Sheffield, Kelso et al., 1978	20
Melbourne, Wood et al., 1981	11

Perinatal mortality rates for each of the trials. Those in white were the "low risk" trials, grey were the "mixed and unknown risk" trials, and those in black were the "high risk" trials

Right at the bottom are the two "low risk" trials, with death rates of 11 and 20 per 10,000 births. And right at the top are two of the "high risk" trials, with death rates of 450 and 1,423 per 10,000. So far, so good. The actual chance of death in these studies lines up with the label they have been given.

But in the middle bit of the table, things are rather messy. There are four studies that have a mortality rate in the 20's. One of these is a "low risk" trial, one is a "mixed risk" trial, and the remaining two were "high risk" trials. You can see it is possible to have more-or-less the same mortality rate, but for the women in that study to be classified as either "low", "mixed", or "high" risk. And if you compare the mortality rate in the Dallas 1986 trial with the mortality rate in the 1976 Denver trial, we have the odd situation of a "mixed risk" trial having a mortality rate that is four times higher than a "high risk" trial.

Trying to predict future outcomes on the basis of the presence or absence of something on a list of risk factors is very inexact. That was clearly the case during the thirty-year time span when the research was done. It remains true today that risk assessment involves a large amount of guess work. There's just so much messiness in what the word "risk" means in this body of research, and in clinical practice, that I think it is better if we don't split the research up this way.

Some additional thoughts about the results for neonatal seizures

I want to include some more thoughts about what the research had to say about neonatal seizures. In arguments in favour of CTG use, the lower seizure rate is often put forward, and sometimes it is used to suggest that all the other outcomes are also better with CTG use, but we just haven't done the right research to prove it (Royal Australian and New Zealand College of Obstetrics and Gynaecology, 2019). So I think it is a good idea to look more closely to decide just how confident to be with the statement that CTG use prevents neonatal seizures.

Here's the first thing that stands out for me. If all the ways that brain injury shows up in babies are caused by the same thing – low oxygen levels – and the way that CTG monitoring is meant to work is the same for each of these outcomes, then you would expect to see that the numbers of brain injury related conditions was lower in the CTG monitored group across all the outcomes. The same direction and size of change in outcome should be visible even if the studies weren't big enough for the difference to be statistically significant.

You would therefore expect that with rates of seizures with CTG use, there would also be lower rates of cerebral palsy, even if the size of the studies means this difference was not statistically significant. Two trials looked at both neonatal seizures and cerebral palsy rates – the Dublin trial and the preterm birth trial done in Seattle (Grant et al., 1989; Luthy et l., 1987; MacDonald et al., 1985; Shy et al., 1990). The Dublin trial found a 55% reduction in seizures but a 20% higher rate of cerebral palsy with CTG use. The preterm birth trial found no difference in seizure rates, but a 254% *increase* in cerebral palsy with CTG use. So the theory that CTG monitoring must make outcomes other than seizures better too, but the research wasn't powerful enough to show it, doesn't add up here.

The authors of the paper presenting the long term follow up from the Dublin trial (Grant et al., 1989) noted the difference in their findings and suggested some ideas about why there was a lower rate of seizures but more cases of cerebral palsy. They had three ideas:

1. The kinds of seizures prevented by CTG use are not caused by low oxygen levels – though they thought this was unlikely.

2. The pattern of low oxygen levels that causes seizures is different to the pattern of low oxygen levels that cause cerebral palsy.

3. Cerebral palsy that happens to babies who had seizures soon after birth is not due to low oxygen levels.

Researchers haven't really sorted out the answer to this confusing picture in the years since the study was published.

People should therefore be really cautious about making the assumption that the reduction in neonatal seizures is a clue that CTG monitoring works for all sorts of other things but we haven't done enough research to prove it.

Neonatal seizures and the use of oxytocin during labour

The other bit of detail I want to share with you about neonatal seizures is tucked away deep inside the fine print of the Dublin trial (MacDonald et al., 1985). The authors don't actually mention this in the paper itself, and I needed to do a bit of maths using the numbers they provided to produce this summary for you. This bit of information helps to suggest a group of women whose babies might do well with CTG monitoring and a group whose babies don't appear to benefit at all from it.

There's a table in the paper (Table XIV on page 535) where they start with the group of babies who had neonatal seizures, split them up according to whether their mothers were in the CTG monitoring or intermittent auscultation groups, and then split them up again according to whether oxytocin was given during their mother's labour (for induction or to speed up a slow labour) or not. Using the numbers from this table I was able to calculate and compare the rates of seizures in these four groups:

✧ When oxytocin was used during labour and the woman was in the intermittent auscultation group, the rate of neonatal seizures was 160 per 10,000 births.

✧ When oxytocin was used during labour and the woman was in the CTG monitoring group, the rate of neonatal seizures was 36 in 10,000 births – the difference between the two types of monitoring is statistically significant.

Next –

✧ When oxytocin was not used during labour and the woman was in the CTG monitoring group, the rate of neonatal seizures was 21 per 10,000 births.

✧ When oxytocin was not used during labour and the woman was in the intermittent auscultation group, the rate of neonatal seizures was *also* 21 per 10,000 births. You don't need a fancy statistics calculator to recognise that this was not significantly different from the CTG monitoring group.

What do these numbers tell us about this study? First, when oxytocin was used, more babies had neonatal seizures. Second, CTG monitoring when oxytocin was being used didn't bring the seizure rate down to the same level as when it wasn't being used. Extra risk from using oxytocin was still present. And finally, when oxytocin wasn't in use, the rate of neonatal seizures was no different between CTG use and intermittent auscultation.

Are the findings about oxytocin use still relevant today?

While CTG use seemed to be a better option for women who were being given oxytocin in this study from the early 1980s, does that mean it is *still* a better option for women using oxytocin to have CTG monitoring for their labour today? Another paper published by some of the same research team, in the same year as the Dublin trial (Garcia et al., 1985), gives some more insight into how maternity care was delivered to women during the period of the trial and how it differs from today. They said that (p. 80):

> Each woman is assigned a companion, usually a student midwife, but sometimes a medical student, who remains with her throughout labor, monitors her progress and, most importantly, encourages and supports her. Overall responsibility for the delivery suite is in the hands of a senior midwife to whom those giving immediate care will turn if they are concerned and who will, herself, seek the advice of a senior obstetrician if necessary.

The other bit of detail that isn't in the paper is the precise way that oxytocin was given in the Dublin trial. Nowadays, an infusion pump is used – an electronic device that attaches to the tubing of an intravenous infusion set and can be programmed to give a very precise dose of fluid per minute. At the time of the Dublin trial these were not in use. Instead, infusion rates would be controlled by counting the numbers of drops of liquid that fell through a small chamber in the infusion set and adjusting the rate up and down by rolling a small plastic wheel that either squeezed the tubing more tightly, or released the tubing a bit. These manual adjustments were never as accurate as can now be achieved with infusion pumps, which is why infusion pumps are now routinely used whenever medications that require precise dosing are used.

What was happening at the time of the Dublin trial was that medical and midwifery students were left pretty much on their own to manually adjust the oxytocin rate until enough, but not too many, contractions were happening. This would now be considered dangerous and unprofessional practice. A student would no longer be left alone to independently manage a woman's care, only asking for help when they felt they should. And no one would deliver oxytocin these days without an infusion pump to control the rate.

Current approaches to providing care to women when oxytocin is in use have made an impact on the outcomes of that care. The rate of seizures seen in the Dublin trial for women where oxytocin was used was much higher than are seen in current practice. In the ARRIVE trial that tested whether or not it is better to induce women having their first baby at 39 weeks of pregnancy (Grobman et al., 2018; and all women in this trial will almost certainly have had CTG monitoring), the rate of seizures in the group being induced early was 4 in 10,000 – not 36 per 10,000 as was the case in the Dublin trial.

> Because the way women are cared for when oxytocin is in use during labour is now very different to the way that they were cared for during the Dublin trial, it means that we can't safely cut-and-paste the findings of the Dublin trial into current practice. It might be that CTG use is still associated with a lower seizure rate for women using oxytocin. Or it might be that there is no longer an association at all. We simply don't know.

I think it is therefore reasonable to be hesitant about making claims that using CTG monitoring for a woman's labour today in a high-income country will reduce her chance of her baby developing seizures after birth.

Outcomes for women

Now that we have looked in detail at what the research had to say about outcomes for babies, let's turn to what the research had to say about outcomes for the women in the trials. This is important, because each women who is making decisions about which type of fetal heart rate monitoring approach will want to decide how to balance any advantages and disadvantages in outcomes for themselves, as well as for their babies.

How women gave birth

The Cochrane review includes information about caesarean section from eleven trials between 1976 and 2006, that included 18,861 women (Alfirevic et al., 2017). For instrumental birth (forceps and vacuum), it includes ten trials over the same time period with 18,615 women providing data. There was a statistically significant increase in the caesarean section rate in the CTG monitoring group. There was also a higher rate of instrumental births. If you look at only the caesarean sections and instrumental births done because of concerns about the health of the fetus, once again there was a higher rate of both in women in the CTG monitoring group.

No statistically significant differences were found in the Cochrane review (Alfirevic et al., 2017) for:

✧ The use of epidural pain relief in labour

✧ The use of other drugs for pain relief in labour

✧ The use of oxytocin (used to speed labour up).

Does "risk" make a difference here too?

Let's now look at how the results break down according to risk for outcomes for women (Alfirevic et al., 2017). For women considered to be "low risk", caesarean section rates were higher when CTG monitoring was used and there was no statistically significant difference in the instrumental birth rate. Adding these together to get the rate of surgical birth, there was a statistically significant difference, with surgical birth being more common in the CTG monitoring group.

Surgical birth rates were also statistically significantly higher for women allocated to CTG monitoring in the "mixed" and "high risk" studies, but the type of birth that made the difference changed. In the "mixed risk" studies, there was no difference in the caesarean section rate but more instrumental births in the CTG monitoring group. In the high-risk population, the caesarean section rate was higher in the CTG monitoring group but there was no difference in instrumental births. The higher rate of surgical birth was consistent across all the risk categories (an increase of around 22%).

In summary, CTG monitoring was associated with higher rates of surgical birth across all the risk groups.

"But I have (this specific risk factor). What does the research say about it?"

I am often asked questions like: What does the evidence say about CTG monitoring for women planning a vaginal birth after caesarean section? What does the evidence say for women over the age of 40? What does the evidence say about women who are being induced? To answer questions like this, researchers would need to include only women planning vaginal birth after caesarean section, or only women over the age of 40, or only women being induced, then randomly split them up so that some have CTG monitoring, and the remainder have intermittent auscultation so comparisons could be made between the two monitoring options.

That isn't the way that most of the research was done, however. The majority of the trials that included women considered to be a "high risk" included anyone with one or more of anything from a long list of risk factors. It is impossible to dig into the fine print of the paper and see whether the babies of women with (name your chosen specific risk factor) do better with CTG use than they do with intermittent auscultation or not. In theory at least, it might be that babies born to women with risk factor A have much better outcomes with CTG use, and that babies born to women with risk factor B do much better with intermittent auscultation, but when you smoosh the results together, you can no longer see the difference.

There have been three trials that looked at women who all had just the one same risk factor. These trials looked at women who were in preterm labour, who had meconium-stained amniotic fluid, or who were planning a vaginal birth after one previous caesarean section. I'll quickly summarise each of them.

Preterm labour

All the women in this trial were in preterm labour, between 26 and 32 weeks of pregnancy, or with a baby who was expected to weigh between 750 and 1,700 grams (when the due date was not certain) (Luthy et al., 1987; Shy et al., 1990). 246 women participated in the trial, with 173 babies followed through until they were 18 months old. This trial found no difference in mortality rates or neonatal seizures, but higher rates of caesarean section and a much higher rate of cerebral palsy in the group who were allocated to CTG monitoring. It is important to note this was a small trial, so I would suggest being cautious about saying that CTG monitoring in preterm labour is linked to cerebral palsy without more research to double check what they found. *It surprises me that in the decades since this research was done, no research group has set out to do exactly that.*

Meconium-stained amniotic fluid

Meconium is the name given to the first bowel motion (poo) that babies do. Sometimes the baby opens its bowel before birth so meconium mixes into the fluid that surrounds the baby, called amniotic fluid or liquor. Depending on the amount of amniotic fluid and the amount of meconium in it, meconium-stained amniotic fluid can be seen as a very vague green tinge, or it can look like thick pea soup.

There are several reasons a fetus might pass meconium before birth. One of these is low oxygen supply. Meconium-stained amniotic fluid, particularly when it is thick, is therefore considered a sign that the fetus has a higher chance of low oxygen levels during labour. Research confirms babies who had meconium-stained amniotic fluid were more likely to have complications after birth (Argyridis & Arulkumaran, 2016).

One of the fetal heart rate monitoring trials looked at women with meconium-staining of the amniotic fluid. This was an unpublished study done in Pakistan in 1989. There is a little bit of information about this study in the Cochrane review (Alfirevic et al., 2017). 200 women were included. There were no differences in mortality rates, or instrumental births, but higher rates of caesarean section with CTG use. They didn't provide data about neonatal seizures. Again, this study was too small to be really useful.

Vaginal birth after caesarean section

There is a small increase in the chance of stillbirth during labour or death of the baby in the first week of life when women plan to have a vaginal birth when they have previously given birth by caesarean section. The chance of this outcome in a recent large study from Scotland was 7 in 10,000 with planned vaginal birth (Fitzpatrick, et al., 2019). Because of this, women planning vaginal birth after caesarean section are considered to be at higher risk and are recommended to have CTG monitoring.

One trial has looked at this, with 100 women taking part (Madaan & Trivedi, 2006). All had one previous caesarean section, and 54 of the women had also had a vaginal birth before or after their caesarean section. No deaths occurred during the study and the authors didn't look at neonatal seizures. The caesarean section rate was higher in women in the CTG monitoring group but due to the small size of the study, this wasn't statistically significant. Again, the small size of this study means we can't rely on this to tell us what is the better approach for women who have previously given birth by caesarean section.

Answers from other types of research

One of the major drawbacks to the research from the randomised controlled trials is that it is quite old. The other issue is that even when you add all the studies together, the total number of babies included is not big enough to provide high levels of confidence in the accuracy of the results, particularly for things like stillbirth during labour which is fortunately very rare. It has been calculated that at least 360,000 women would need to be included in the trials to be considered big enough to produce reliable results (Thompson, 1981). Other types of research have looked at the question of which approach to fetal monitoring was best and this research is more recent. While these types of research are not considered to be as reliable as randomised controlled trials, they do help to add to the overall picture of what is known about fetal heart rate monitoring options.

One research team (Heelan-Fancher et al., 2019) used data collected in the USA from over one million women considered to be low-risk at the start of labour. Some women had intermittent auscultation and others had CTG monitoring. Unlike the randomised controlled trials, the decision about which type of monitoring to use was not randomly determined but was chosen by the woman or her maternity professional. Factors that the researchers knew might impact on the outcomes but had nothing to do with the type of monitoring (like whether this was the woman's first birth, how old she was, and what the baby weighed at birth) were taken into account through mathematical means so they were less likely to confuse the results.

The researchers found the mortality rate in babies who were monitored in labour by CTG monitoring was no different to when intermittent auscultation was used. There was also no difference in the Apgar score at five minutes of age. What did change was the rate of caesarean section and instrumental birth, with both being more common for women who had CTG monitoring.

Together with my supervisors, one of the things I looked at during my doctoral studies was evidence from studies other than randomised controlled trials done in groups of women considered to be at higher risk by the standards of the time (Small et al., 2020). We thoroughly searched databases to identify any research about the use of CTG monitoring in high-risk populations. We found 27 studies, published between 1972 and 2018. Having found the research papers, the next step was to look at whether the research was done in a way that meant that the results were likely to be due to something other than the type of fetal heart rate monitoring that was used during labour. We used a research tool called the Risk of Bias in Nonrandomised Studies of Interventions (Sterne et al., 2016). According to the creators of the tool, studies that are at critical or high risk of bias should not be relied on to give useful evidence on which to base practice, while those at moderate and low risk are suitable for this use. Of the 27 studies, five were at moderate risk and none at low risk for bias.

These five moderate-risk studies were published between 1978 and 2018. They ranged in size from 235 to 1.2 million women. None looked at long term brain injury. The studies showed no difference in the rates of stillbirth or neonatal death between CTG monitoring and intermittent auscultation during labour.

The findings from these other types of research reflect the findings seen in the randomised controlled trials, suggesting that despite improved CTG technology, better education of maternity professionals, and better systems of care, we still haven't been able to make CTG monitoring live up to our hopes and dreams for it.

How I think these research results should be used

As a researcher, I love playing about with research findings simply for the joy of learning new things and thinking about what they mean. But the main reason fetal monitoring research has been done is to try to make things better for women and their babies when they use maternity services. So, here is my *opinion* (based on deep understanding of the research) on how I think we should best make use of the research findings in clinical practice.

I think that the whole idea of "risk" as it plays out in fetal monitoring research and in practice is a great big pile of mess. Because of that, we should not split the research up into risk categories. I believe the research findings should be combined for analysis, as this gives the biggest numbers and therefore provides the most robust findings that are possible from the existing evidence. When you do that, I see nothing in the results that convince me that using CTG monitoring in labour can offer a reduction in the death rate or in the cerebral palsy rate, and I don't have much confidence that the differences seen in seizure rates apply in today's maternity care settings. I can also see that women are generally worse off with CTG monitoring – something I'll explore more in the next chapter.

In summary – it is my opinion that CTGs don't work for babies and they harm some women.

I also believe we should not advise different fetal monitoring approaches for women according to their risk category. ALL women should be given information about the options available and what the research says, be supported as they make a decision (never coerced or manipulated), and have their decisions respected.

What about admission CTGs?

Before I finish up this chapter that has looked at what research says about the comparison between CTG monitoring and intermittent auscultation in labour, I want to include two short sections about other ways that CTG monitoring is used. The first is what is known as an admission CTG.

Admission CTGs involve a short (usually about 30 minutes) period of CTG monitoring when a woman first arrives at a maternity service in labour, before continuing on with intermittent auscultation for the labour. Admission CTGs are used commonly in some places, and not in others. They are typically used for women considered as "low risk", as the expectation is that women considered to be at "high risk" will begin with and then continue with CTG monitoring for the duration of their labour. Women who have anything other than a normal fetal heart rate pattern detected on the admission CTG recording are then advised to keep going with CTG monitoring in labour, in the belief that this can prevent a poor outcome. In some women, the heart rate pattern will be sufficiently abnormal that immediate birth by caesarean section might be advised.

> The main flaw in the argument in favour of admission CTG monitoring is easy to spot. For it to work in the way people think it does, then using continuous CTG monitoring in labour would need to improve outcomes for the fetus / baby. As you have just seen, there's no convincing proof that it does.

Nonetheless, let's look at what the research says rather than just making assumptions.

There have been five randomised controlled trials that provide evidence about admission CTG monitoring. All have been done with women considered to be "low risk". The first four trials were summarised in a Cochrane review (Devane, et al., 2017). The most recent trial was published after that review (Smith, et al., 2018) and therefore wasn't included. I have added the outcomes for the new trial to the previous ones, so you have all the evidence summarised together.

The studies were published between 2001 and 2018, so the evidence is more recent than we have for using CTG monitoring continuously during labour. In total, 14,373 women were included. The perinatal mortality rate was not statistically different between women randomly allocated to admission CTG and those allocated to intermittent auscultation. There was also no difference in the incidence of hypoxic-ischaemic encephalopathy. Neonatal seizures were not reported in the studies, and no long-term follow-up has been performed to know if the type of monitoring made a difference to cerebral palsy rates.

There were no statistically significant differences in the use of caesarean section or instrumental birth. The rate of continuous CTG monitoring was high in both groups, at 62% for those allocated to an admission CTG and 48% for those allocated to intermittent auscultation.

The number of women included in research about admission CTGs was less than the number of women in research about continuous CTG monitoring in labour. It is theoretically possible that there might be a difference in outcomes for the baby that would become visible if more women were included in research. However, it seems improbable to me given the way that admission CTG monitoring is meant to work and what we know about continuous CTG use.

What about CTG use during pregnancy?

Antenatal CTG monitoring refers to the use of CTG monitoring during pregnancy. It is typically used when there is something clearly not right (an episode of bleeding) or when women are considered to be at higher risk for a problem relating to the wellbeing of their baby (like being "overdue"). Antenatal CTG monitoring generally involves recording the fetal heart rate for about 20 to 30 minutes, or however long it takes to achieve set criteria that define the heart rate pattern as normal.

Researchers have investigated whether antenatal CTG monitoring changes outcomes for women and their babies, with the findings in a Cochrane review (Grivell et al., 2015). There have been four randomised controlled trials, published between 1982 and 1985, with the number of women in each trial ranging from 300 to 539. All the women in the trials were considered to be higher risk – including things like pre-eclampsia, a suspected small baby, and being "overdue".

How the research was done was clearly described in three of the trials, but the other was a bit vague. In the three well-described studies, all the women had a CTG trace. Half of them had the CTG trace interpreted and used to guide decisions about their care. The other half had the CTG put into a sealed envelope that was only opened after the birth of their baby.

The perinatal mortality rate was 230 per 10,000 births in the group where the CTG information was used and 110 per 10,000 births in the group where it was not used. The difference here gets close to being statistically significant but does not quite make it. There were no differences in the rates of neonatal seizures, Apgar scores, admissions to the neonatal unit, or in the number of weeks of pregnancy when women gave birth. There were also no differences in the use of induction of labour or caesarean section.

I find it worrying that 40 years ago researchers never got around to fully investigating what was going on here. Does using CTGs during pregnancy really increase the chance of the baby dying, or not? We don't actually know for sure.

Summary

Intermittent auscultation produced the same results as CTG monitoring when it came to how many babies were lost to stillbirth during labour, or the death of the baby in the first week of life, and this was true across all risk categories. Women in the CTG monitoring group had less chance of their baby having seizures after birth, with one less baby being affected for every 667 women who had CTG monitoring rather than intermittent auscultation. Due to significant changes in the way care is provided during labour, I suspect that using CTG monitoring for a woman's labour today would not achieve the same outcome. Overall, cerebral palsy rates were the same whether CTG monitoring or intermittent auscultation was used.

CTG monitoring was associated with higher rates of surgical birth across all the risk groups.

The findings from recent, good quality research other than randomised controlled trials reflects the findings seen in the randomised controlled trials, suggesting that despite improved CTG technology, better education of maternity professionals, and better systems of care, CTG monitoring still doesn't deliver the kinds of outcomes many believe that it does.

I believe it is important that all women should be given information during pregnancy about the various options for fetal heart rate monitoring so they can weigh up that information and make their mind up about what they will, or will not use, during their pregnancy and for their labour.

While I have touched on some of the downsides of each fetal heart rate monitoring approach, there is more information to consider that could be useful for your decision making. That's what you will find in the next chapter.

CHAPTER 5

What are the downsides?

When making decisions, a common approach is to weigh up the chance of benefit against the chance of harm. The evidence covered in the last chapter helps with this process but there are additional harms to consider that haven't been assessed well (or at all) in randomised controlled trials. In this chapter, I'll take you through other research that explores possible harms of each fetal monitoring approach. Primarily my focus in this chapter is on things of importance to women and families, but I also include a discussion at the end of the chapter about the benefit / harm balance as it works out for maternity care systems. Because the outcomes that affect women are usually more common than the outcomes about babies, the numbers I will give you for women are based every 1,000 women giving birth, while for babies the outcomes are based on every 10,000 babies born.

Harms from intermittent auscultation

As explained in the last chapter, women who have intermittent auscultation in labour rather than using CTG monitoring were slightly more likely to give birth to a baby who has neonatal seizures in the days after birth. This chance was higher among women who had oxytocin used during their labour. Whether these research results are still relevant today is debatable.

Checking the fetal heart rate every 15 minutes, or more often, can disturb a woman who doesn't like frequent physical contact, is trying to sleep, use a bath or birth pool or the shower, or is in a position that requires her to move so the maternity professional can listen to the fetal heart rate.

No other potential harms from intermittent auscultation have been reported in research.

Harms from CTG monitoring

Discomfort and anxiety

Some women describe the straps used to hold sensors in place for CTG monitoring as restrictive and uncomfortable (Smith et al., 2017). CTG monitoring can produce a "technical atmosphere" in the birth room, leading partners and health practitioners to focus on the monitor, rather than on the birthing woman. Women also described anxiety about how the technology worked (for example women feared that they might be electrocuted by it) and changes in the fetal heart rate generated anxiety about whether their fetus was "distressed" (Smith et al., 2017).

There has been research exploring whether there is a relationship between anxiety and CTG monitoring, but it focussed on the use of CTG monitoring before rather than during labour. Mancuso et al. (2008) used validated tests for anxiety and found a significant increase in anxiety scores after CTG monitoring in pregnancy. Many years prior to this, Shalev et al. (1985) compared blood levels of hormones associated with stress in a group of women exposed to CTG monitoring during pregnancy, and a group without CTG monitoring. A significant rise in women's insulin, cortisol, growth hormone, and catecholamines started 10 minutes after CTG monitoring was begun, with the rise lasting over an hour. We don't know whether the same thing happens in labour.

How women give birth

The largest and most impactful set of potential harms from CTG monitoring relates to more frequent use of caesarean section and instrumental birth. As we saw in the last chapter, these are both more common when CTG monitoring is used. Caesarean section or instrumental birth can be seen as simply another way to give birth, but they can also be viewed as harmful if these were not the way the woman wanted to give birth. This is particularly the case if they are used when there is no benefit for the fetus / baby or the woman giving birth (Wendland, 2007). Potential harms include things that happen soon after birth, or that can occur many years later; and can affect either the woman or her baby.

Outcomes for women who give birth by caesarean section

Looking at research investigating health outcomes among women who gave birth by caesarean section, we begin to see why more caesarean sections can be said to be harmful to women. The research looking at harms from caesarean section is recent and reflects current practices that have made caesarean section safer than it was when the randomised controlled trials about fetal heart rate monitoring in labour were done. Most of the research I include here comes from studies comparing planned caesarean section before labour with vaginal birth, rather than unplanned caesarean section done during labour. The chance of a complication happening is higher when caesarean section is done during labour, so these numbers represent a "best case" situation. When the research compared unplanned caesarean birth with vaginal birth, I will make a specific mention of this.

Women who gave birth by caesarean section were more likely to have one of these short-term problems compared to women who had a vaginal birth without the assistance of vacuum or forceps:

✧ Infection (Bodner et al., 2010; Dahlquist et al., 2022; Hammad et al., 2013). This includes having a fever after birth (180 extra women per

1,000), developing a wound infection (79 extra women per 1,000), developing an infection in the uterus called endometritis (three extra women per 1,000), developing a urinary tract infection (three extra women per 1,000), or a breast infection called mastitis (24 extra women per 1,000).

✧ Loss of more than 500 mL of blood after birth, also called postpartum haemorrhage (an extra 68 women per 1,000) (Bodner et al., 2010).

✧ A potentially life-threatening blood clot in the lungs known as pulmonary embolism (0.3 extra women per 1,000) (Dahlquist et al., 2022).

✧ Breastfeeding difficulties (79 extra women per 1,000) (Bodner et al., 2010).

✧ Readmission to hospital because of complications after the birth (11 extra women per 1,000) (Declercq et al., 2007).

✧ Death (0.4 – 0.8 extra women per 1,000) (Esteves-Pereira et al., 2016; Fahmy et al., 2018; Mascarello et al., 2017).

Women who gave birth by caesarean section were also more likely to have one of these long-term outcomes:

✧ Painful sex (six months after giving birth an extra 100 women per 1,000 when comparing unplanned caesarean section in labour with vaginal birth with no tearing) (McDonald et al., 2015).

✧ Complications in their next pregnancy (Keag et al., 2018). I have not been able to find numbers that help us to understand how often these happen for most of these. The problems that were more common were difficulty becoming pregnant, miscarriage, ectopic pregnancy, stillbirth, problems with the placement of the placenta that can cause heavy bleeding, rupture of the uterus (this happens for about two women in every 1,000 who go into labour after having had one previous caesarean section) (Dekker et al., 2010), and needing to have the uterus removed (hysterectomy) soon after birth because of heavy bleeding that was not able to be controlled with the usual treatments.

✧ Scarring from the caesarean surgery. This makes later uterine surgery more challenging. Complications after a hysterectomy done later in life, for example as a treatment for heavy periods, are more common (Lindquist et al., 2017). Surgical complications affected an extra 21 women per 1,000 who had previously had one caesarean section, and 18 extra women per 1,000 had a second operation for those complications.

Outcomes for women who had an instrumental birth

Instrumental birth (forceps and vacuum) was used more often for women allocated to CTG monitoring in the randomised controlled trials. Short- and long-term complications for women from the use of forceps or vacuum extraction include:

✧ Injury to the muscles in the woman's anus, called severe perineal trauma or obstetric anal sphincter injury (also called OASI) (Ampt et al., 2015). Compared to women having a non-instrumental vaginal birth without an episiotomy (a cut in the vaginal opening to make it bigger), 60 to 80 extra women per 1,000 who gave birth with forceps and without an episiotomy had severe perineal trauma. For vacuum extraction with an episiotomy the difference was an extra 30 to 40 women per 1,000.

✧ Major damage to the woman's main pelvic floor muscle, called a levator ani defect. This is an issue that has started to be understood in the last 15 years and is best detected by an ultrasound examination. Compared to women who had a non-instrumental vaginal birth, 360 extra women out of every 1,000 who had a forceps birth because of concerns about the fetal heart rate and who had been pushing for less than an hour developed a levator ani defect (Kearney et al., 2010).

✧ Painful sex six months after the baby was born. This happened for an extra 210 women per 1,000 who had a forceps birth, and an extra 290 women per 1,000 who had a vacuum birth, compared to women who had a vaginal birth without the use of instruments to assist (McDonald et al., 2015).

✧ Prolapse of the vagina, bladder, uterus, or bowel 16 to 24 years after birth. This affected an extra 26 women per 1,000 after forceps birth (V[l]løyhaug et al., 2015).

While these injuries are significant for the women who experience them, fortunately, for the majority of women these short- and long-term complications don't happen. When they do, most can be treated with an expectation of a full recovery.

Outcomes for babies born by caesarean section

The baby is also impacted by how they are born. Short term consequences for babies of caesarean birth include:

✧ Injury to the fetus. This affected 16 babies in every 1,000 caesarean sections. Usually this is a small cut and heals well (Hammad et al., 2013).

✧ Jaundice (ten extra babies per 1,000 born by unplanned caesarean section in labour rather than vaginal birth) (Peters et al., 2018).

✧ Feeding problems (20 extra babies per 1,000 born by unplanned caesarean section in labour rather than vaginal birth) (Peters et al., 2018).

✧ Low temperature (ten extra babies per 1,000 born by unplanned caesarean section in labour rather than vaginal birth) (Peters et al., 2018).

Longer term consequences of caesarean birth for the baby include:

✧ Higher rates of conditions affecting the lungs (Slabuszewska-Jozwiak et al., 2020), including -

  · Lung infection (41 extra babies per 1,000 born by caesarean section rather than vaginal birth).

  · Asthma (one extra baby per 1,000 born by caesarean section rather than vaginal birth).

✧ Infections other than in the lungs (20 extra babies per 1,000 born by unplanned caesarean section in labour rather than vaginal birth) (Peters et al., 2018).

- Obesity in childhood (32 extra babies per 1,000 born by caesarean section rather than vaginal birth) (Slabuszewska-Jozwiak et al., 2020).

- Problems with high or low blood sugar, including diabetes (64 extra babies per 1,000 born by unplanned caesarean section in labour rather than vaginal birth (Peters et al., 2018).

- A skin rash called eczema (51 extra babies per 1,000 born by unplanned caesarean section in labour rather than vaginal birth) (Peters et al., 2018).

- Problems with the immune system such as systemic connective tissue disorders, juvenile arthritis, inflammatory bowel disease, immune deficiencies, and leukaemia (Sevelsted et al., 2015) - but there was not enough information provided in the paper to calculate the number of babies affected.

- Neurological disorders leading to hospitalisation. This included autism, eating disorders, and movement disorders (six extra babies per 1,000 born by caesarean section rather than vaginal birth) (Baumfeld et al., 2018).

- Learning problems in childhood affecting reading, writing, number skills, and so on (Polidano et al., 2017). There was not enough information provided in the paper to calculate the number affected.

Outcomes for babies born by instrumental birth

Short term problems related to instrumental birth described in research are:

- Jaundice (50 extra babies per 1,000 born with either forceps or vacuum rather than after non-instrumental vaginal birth) (Peters et al., 2018).

- Feeding problems (20 extra babies per 1,000 born with either forceps or vacuum rather than after non-instrumental vaginal birth) (Peters et al., 2018).

- Cuts or bruises on the scalp occurring in 100 of 1,000 of births by vacuum extraction (Doumouchtsis & Arulkumaran, 2006).

✧ Bleeding into the scalp skin occurring in 60 of 1,000 of births by vacuum extraction, and also more common after forceps birth than non-instrumental vaginal birth (Doumouchtsis & Arulkumaran, 2006).

✧ Skull fractures. These are rare but can occur with both forceps and vacuum instruments (Doumouchtsis & Arulkumaran, 2006).

✧ Bleeding in the outside layers of the brain (subdural or cerebral haemorrhage) occurring in an extra 0.5 babies per 1,000 born with vacuum, and an 0.7 extra per 1,000 born with forceps, compared with non-instrumental vaginal birth (Doumouchtsis & Arulkumaran, 2006).

✧ Bleeding deep in the brain (subarachnoid haemorrhage) occurring in an extra 0.1 per 1,000 babies born with vacuum, and an extra 0.2 per 1,000 with forceps, compared with non-instrumental vaginal birth (Doumouchtsis & Arulkumaran, 2006).

✧ Eye injuries occurring at a rate of approximately two per 1,000 after forceps birth (McAnena et al., 2015).

✧ Shoulder dystocia (when the baby's shoulders become stuck against the bones of the woman's pelvis and extra steps are needed to release them) occurring in an extra 21 babies per 1,000 born with vacuum, and at a similar rate with forceps, compared with non-instrumental vaginal birth (Asta et al., 2016).

✧ When shoulder dystocia occurs, nerve injury occurs in an extra 130 babies of 1,000 with shoulder dystocia after forceps, and an extra 40 per 1,000 born with shoulder dystocia after vacuum, compared with shoulder dystocia occurring after non-instrumental vaginal birth (Brimacombe et al., 2008).

Longer term problems after instrumental birth have not been as comprehensively researched as they have been for caesarean section. This is what we know:

✧ Eczema after instrumental birth affects an extra 41 babies per 1,000, compared with non-instrumental vaginal birth (Peters et al., 2018)

✧ Asthma affects an extra 100 babies per 1,000 after forceps birth, compared with non-instrumental vaginal birth (Hancox et al., 2013)

While most women and their babies will not experience a complication relating to the use of caesarean section or instrumental birth, some will. When the use of CTG monitoring leads to little to no improvement in other outcomes, these complications are therefore not balanced out by benefits.

Harms from fetal spiral electrodes and intrauterine pressure catheters

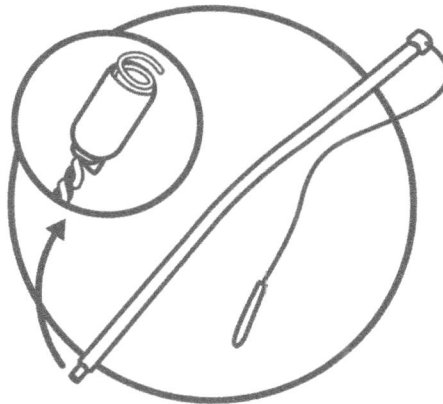

Fetal spiral electrode with a close-up of the tip that attaches to the fetus

Internal CTG monitoring has been associated with specific complications that don't happen with external monitoring. The use of a fetal spiral electrode has been associated with damage to the fetal scalp. An extra three in 1,000 babies born vaginally without the assistance of vacuum or forceps who had a fetal spiral electrode had visible scalp injuries compared to those who did not have a fetal spiral electrode (Kawakita et al., 2016). Babies were also marginally more likely to have bleeding under the skin of the scalp (cephalohaematoma) – an additional one per 1,000 (Kawakita et al., 2016). Although rare, this can lead to the baby developing jaundice (D'souza et al., 1982). Serious skin infections can develop at the site where the scalp clip was attached (Davey & Moore, 2006; Hsieh et al., 1999; Siddiqi & Taylor, 1982), and this can spread to the brain (Fick & Woerdeman, 2021) or into the blood causing sepsis (Kawakita et al., 2016).

Women were more likely to develop a fever during labour (17 more per 1,000), or after birth (19 more per 1,000), when a fetal spiral electrode was used (Kawakita et al., 2016). They were also more likely to be diagnosed with infection in the uterus during labour (chorioamnionitis – an extra 26 per 1000), or after birth (endometritis – an extra seven per 1,000) (Kawakita et al., 2016).

The use of intrauterine pressure catheters has been associated with a potentially serious complication called uterine perforation where the tip of the catheter makes a hole in the wall of the uterus (Chan et al., 1973; Rood, 2012). Accurate numbers for how often this complication occurs have not been published. Fever during labour was more common when intrauterine pressure monitoring was used, occurring in 6 – 14% of women rather than 2 - 5% when it was not used (Frolova et al., 2021; Harper et al., 2013).

> While the chances of a complication when using these monitoring devices is small and may be minimised by good technique and giving preventative antibiotics (which have their own potential problems), complications from internal monitoring equipment can be avoided by using either intermittent auscultation or external CTG monitoring.

Abnormal heart rate patterns?

As previously described, the very first randomised controlled trial (Haverkamp et al., 1976) used an interesting approach for their research that hasn't been repeated since. All the women in the study had internal CTG monitoring, but those who were randomly chosen for the intermittent auscultation group had the CTG recording hidden from view so it could not be used during labour to guide decision making. A nurse regularly listened to the fetal heart and this information was used instead. This approach meant that there was a CTG recording to look at after their babies were born for all the women in the study, not only for those where it was used to guide care during labour.

These researchers found that women in the CTG monitoring group were more likely to have had abnormal fetal heart rate patterns during early labour than women in the intermittent auscultation group. Why this might have happened is an interesting question. The study authors wrote (p. 316):

> Subtle, less obvious factors involved in the actual care of labouring patients could influence infant outcome. The patients who were auscultated had individualised nursing care with one of the project nurses at the bedside almost continually. Very close physical contact with the patient was necessary for the nurse to auscultate fetal heart tones adequately. This was not true to the same degree with the [CTG] monitored group. Nursing attention with respect to maternal comfort, emotional support, and "laying on of hands" could have a significant impact on the fetus. Patients who have a [CTG] monitor adjacent to their bed are often bothered and stressed by flashing light, the sound produced by each fetal heart beat, and hearing or seeing decelerations even when they are benign. The authors have the impression that the reassuring psychological atmosphere created by personal nurse interaction and the absence of the recording machine contributed to the excellent infant outcome in auscultation patients.

This is the only study carried out to date that made it possible to consider whether CTG monitoring might be associated with the development of abnormal fetal heart rate patterns. It raises an important question: *could it be that anxiety because of the presence of the CTG monitor and the relative absence of personalised professional support creates the very problem the CTG monitor was designed to address*? It could also be that what was seen in this study happened by pure chance, so repeating this approach would be useful. Sadly, this has never been done.

Autism?

Theoretical concerns have been raised questioning whether prolonged exposure to Doppler ultrasound as part of continuous CTG monitoring during a long labour might be a risk factor for the development of autism (Rodgers, 2020; 2025). Rodgers looked at the timing of the introduction of CTG monitoring and showed this coincides with a substantial increase in the rate of autism. She noted animal studies that showed that prolonged exposure to ultrasound can impact on the development of the fetal brain.

> Clearly, this is a theory only, and there is currently no research that has either confirmed or denied it.

Fetal exposure to Doppler ultrasound can be reduced by using intermittent auscultation with a handheld Doppler (listening for one minute every 15 minutes means less exposure than listening continuously for 15 minutes) or avoided completely by intermittent auscultation with a Pinard. Using a fetal spiral electrode to record the fetal ECG also avoids Doppler ultrasound but introduces other possible harms at the same time.

CTG monitoring changes the way maternity professionals relate to birthing women

Using CTG monitoring in labour changes the way midwives and the other professionals who provide maternity care work with women in labour and how they work with each other. From the research exploring women's experiences of CTG monitoring (Smith et al., 2017), women reported CTG monitoring introduced a technical and impersonal atmosphere to their labour. When there were issues with the quality of the recording, other clinicians were called into the birth room, producing a lack of privacy. Staff were said to be overly focussed on the CTG machine to the detriment of the woman. Doctors were described as hovering around the monitor, while in other research women reported being left alone by their midwife more often and for longer periods when CTG monitoring was in use (Garcia et al., 1985).

Extra work for maternity professionals

Recent evidence has explored the work labour nurses in the USA needed to do to ensure an interpretable CTG recording was being generated for the entire duration of labour (Fox, A., et al., 2022). While for some women CTG monitoring means they don't have to be touched regularly to determine the fetal heart rate, the findings of this research showed this wasn't always the case. Almost 50% of nurses in this study said they spent 1-2 hours during a 12-hour work shift manipulating CTG sensors and a similar number reported spending 1-2 hours per shift helping women change position to achieve a continuous recording of the fetal heart rate. The authors noted "approximately half of participants spend up to one third of their shifts in efforts to achieve fetal monitoring" (p. 4).

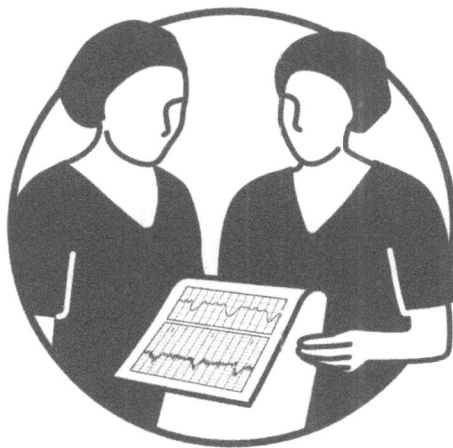

Some people might argue (despite the evidence about CTG monitoring) that adjusting equipment, assisting women to change position, and adding documentation to the CTG is time well invested. There is a downside to this though.

> When maternity professionals are busy with these things there are other things they are not doing. Maternity professionals can't focus on ensuring the safety of the woman and her fetus, meeting her needs for support and encouragement, and communicating with other members of the maternity care team to coordinate treatment, if much of their time and thought space is taken up by work with the CTG equipment.

Potential for understaffing

Given the extra time required to maintain a continuously readable CTG trace, it could be argued that more staff are needed when CTG monitoring is being used. However, sometimes what happens instead is that CTG monitoring is used as a replacement for a maternity professional when there aren't quite enough staff. Many researchers have noted this (Dover & Gauge, 1995; Hindley, et al., 2006; Jepsen, et al 2022; Munro, et al., 2002; Walker, et al., 2001). It has been called "midwife by proxy" or using the CTG machine as a "babysitter".

One midwife in the study by Munro and colleagues said of the CTG machine: "It can be used so you can go out and look after your fourth patient and come back in and see that the baby has been alright at the time you have gone" (2002, p. 497). The problem with this is that without anyone to interpret or act on an abnormal pattern in the CTG, there is no conceivable way that using CTG monitoring will improve outcomes.

> At worst, using the CTG as a "babysitter" might lead to a woman being left alone with no support for prolonged periods of time with no one noting the development of serious complications.

If you choose to use CTG monitoring, and are finding you are left alone at times when you want the support of a maternity professional, here are some options:

✧ Press the call bell and when someone answers, ask that they stay in the room with you.

✧ If no one answers the call bell, have your support partner leave your room and look for a member of staff to ask them to attend the room.

✧ Remove the CTG sensors (NEVER pull off a fetal spiral electrode however!), or disconnect the leads to the CTG machine, or turn off the power to the machine. This works if central fetal monitoring is in use, as someone at the central monitoring station will notice and come to the room to see why the CTG recording suddenly stopped. You can then ask them to ensure a professional stays with you.

Healthcare system downsides

The final "harms" to consider are the downsides for the healthcare system. I have already touched on one aspect of what is known as an "opportunity cost". When you are doing thing A, you can't also be doing thing B. If thing B is what ensures safe outcomes, then spending time or money on thing A, stops you from doing the things needed to achieve safety. So far, we have looked at ways in which CTG monitoring take up time that could be spent doing other things to keep women and their babies safe.

Another opportunity cost relates to the use of limited healthcare resources. Any maternity service has finite resources available at any one point in time. There are only so many CTG machines, so many maternity professionals, so many operating theatres available, and so on. We have seen from the research evidence how using CTG monitoring drives up the caesarean section rate. These caesarean sections are unplanned and because they raise concerns about the wellbeing of the baby, they are usually done as soon as possible.

Each woman having a caesarean section requires specialised care from a team of highly skilled professionals: peri-operative nurses, anaesthetists, anaesthetic nurses, neonatal nurses and doctors, midwives, and obstetricians. This takes place in a designated area in the hospital where surgery is performed – an operating room. When a caesarean section is being done, those people, that room, and all the equipment in it are not available for someone else.

In many places, emergency caesarean sections are done by disrupting a planned surgery list. This can result in people having their surgery cancelled as there was no longer time available in an operating room to do it. The higher the caesarean section rate, the more likely this is to happen, and the longer waiting lists get. This adds to the burden of healthcare suffering.

In some places there is a dedicated team and operating room set aside just for emergency caesarean sections. When this is the case the potential "opportunity cost" is less, though it is not uncommon for multiple women to need access to the one operating theatre at the same time, and decisions must be made about who goes first and who waits. With higher rates of unplanned urgent caesarean section this happens more often.

Money is also finite in healthcare systems. Basic CTG machines cost a fair bit of money. Complex central monitoring systems, with added computer interpretation software, linked to an electronic health care record, requiring a touch screen monitor in each birth room, and a bank of computers and monitor screens at the central monitoring station are very expensive. There are ongoing costs to replace lost or broken equipment and to keep the software updated, for example when CTG interpretation guidelines are updated.

Let me give you an example. INFANT is a computerised CTG interpretation system. The INFANT system was evaluated in a randomised controlled trial conducted in the UK (INFANT Collaborative Group, 2017), with no better outcomes for babies found when compared to standard CTG monitoring systems. Alongside the trial, a cost analysis was undertaken (Schroeder et al., 2020). The INFANT system added an extra £11 to the cost of caring for each woman. While this is not a lot per woman, if every maternity service in the UK were to use the system, it would add *an extra £8.5 million* or so to the national cost of healthcare each year – for no additional benefit.

When a health service decides to invest in fetal monitoring equipment, that money can not go towards something else. Employing maternity professionals, expanding access to midwifery continuity of carer models, investing in staff education, funding research – all these things cost money too.

> While it isn't always a simple "we are having A so you can't have B" equation, something, somewhere ends up not getting funded when money is spent on more CTG monitoring equipment. When the thing that doesn't get funding is something with proven benefits (like midwifery continuity of carer models – Roebuck et al., 2025) women and their babies really miss out.

Conclusion

Some argue CTG monitoring should be used for all or most women as there might be a benefit that has not yet been convincingly proven by the research done so far, and it can't do any harm. *It is clear this argument doesn't hold up.* When compared with intermittent auscultation, CTG monitoring increases the chance of complications happening for women and their babies. By spending time and money on CTG monitoring, we also run the risk that other important things that could improve the safety of maternity care won't get done.

The next argument I commonly see being put forward in support of CTG monitoring is that the technology that is used to generate the CTG is much better now, and that means that CTG monitoring does work. Join me in the next chapter and let's see whether that holds true or not.

CHAPTER 6

The extra bits and the research about them

Over the previous two chapters, I have shown how CTG monitoring has not been proven to improve outcomes and has the potential to cause harm. Despite this evidence, many maternity professionals believe that because of technological advancements in CTG monitoring that this is no longer true. Or they believe that the moment when CTG monitoring will achieve the goals of better outcomes is just around the corner, if only everyone just tried a little harder.

In this chapter I'm going to explore things that have been added to CTG monitoring aiming to make it better. I'll go through what research tells us about whether each of these additional options improves outcomes or not. The first few things I will cover are items that are in common use (depending on where you are in the world) and are considered part of "normal" CTG monitoring. They are fetal spiral electrodes, intrauterine pressure catheter monitors, and telemetry monitoring. Then I'll run through evidence about fetal blood sampling, fetal stimulation, ST segment analysis, central fetal monitoring, and computer interpretation of the CTG recording.

Fetal spiral electrodes

I've mentioned fetal spiral electrodes in the previous chapters. These were the first approach to recording the fetal heart rate in the early days of CTG monitoring. You could argue that historically speaking they are not an add-in to CTG monitoring, the external fetal heart monitor that uses Doppler technology is. However, in current practice, most women will start with external monitoring and a fetal spiral electrode will be advised when there is a particular challenge with monitoring the fetal heart rate. So I'm covering these here as an "extra bit".

Using a fetal spiral electrode reduces the number and duration of periods of time when the fetal heart rate is not being recorded, compared to using an externally worn Doppler heart rate sensor (Cohen et al., 2012; Euliano, 2017). The theory is that CTG monitoring works best when the fetal heart rate is recorded with fewer gaps in the recording. If this is true, then using a fetal spiral electrode might be a better option than an external Doppler sensor.

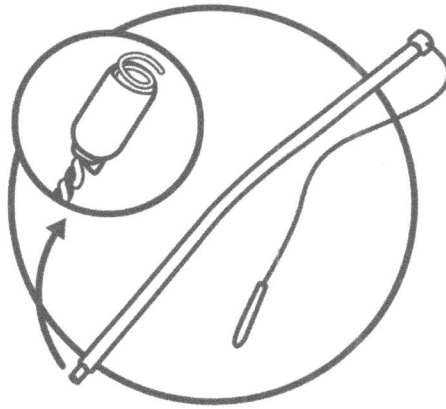

Fetal spiral electrode

Only one study has directly compared the use of a fetal spiral electrode with a Doppler sensor worn externally to generate the CTG recording to see if this translated to benefits for the fetus / baby (Harper et al., 2013). This study was not a randomised controlled trial, and simply looked back to see what was used and what happened. *There has never been a randomised controlled trial that has compared external Doppler sensors with fetal spiral electrodes for gathering fetal heart rate patterns for CTG monitoring.*

In this American research, women who had a fetal spiral electrode for CTG monitoring had longer labours and more vaginal examinations. The caesarean section rate was lower among women who used a fetal spiral electrode. It is possible that women with longer labours were advised to have a fetal spiral electrode, rather than the electrode being somehow responsible for the longer duration of labour. The difference in the caesarean section rate could be due to reduced anxiety on the part of the obstetricians who may have had more confidence in the reliability of the CTG recording when the fetal spiral electrode was in place. There were no differences in Apgar scores, acid levels in the umbilical cord blood, or the number of babies admitted to the neonatal unit when fetal spiral electrodes were used compared with external CTG monitoring.

It is worth noting that in most of the randomised controlled trials about fetal heart rate monitoring in labour discussed in chapter four, fetal spiral electrodes were used. We therefore have evidence comparing the use of fetal spiral electrodes with intermittent auscultation, showing how using a fetal spiral electrode doesn't prevent death or long-term damage to the fetal brain (Alfirevic et al., 2017). Also included in that Cochrane review was one trial that compared continuous CTG use with intermittent CTG use (Herbst & Ingemarsson, 1994). In this study, intermittent CTG use was defined as 15 to 30 minutes of CTG monitoring every second hour, with intermittent auscultation every 15 to 30 minutes when the CTG was not being used. The outcomes for babies in this study was the same, regardless of whether women were randomly assigned to continuous CTG use or intermittent use.

There is therefore no research that shows that capturing every single fetal heart beat with a fetal spiral electrode as part of continuous CTG monitoring is better than selectively capturing information about the fetal heart rate at specific times during a woman's labour. As explained in the last chapter, there is research showing more complications for both women and their babies when fetal spiral electrodes are used rather than other approaches to fetal heart rate monitoring.

Intrauterine pressure catheters for monitoring contractions

Like fetal spiral electrodes, intrauterine pressure monitoring was the original approach to CTG monitoring, but is now typically used only when external monitoring isn't generating a good quality recording. That's why it appears in this chapter as an "extra bit". Maternity professionals in some parts of the world regularly use intrauterine pressure catheters, and in other places they are not used at all. Here in Australia, I have only encountered them once. Check with your maternity care provider whether they are available in the area where you plan to give birth (and your backup facility if relevant) so you know whether you need to have decided on a plan about whether this is something you want or not.

Intrauterine pressure catheters provide more accurate measures of when a woman's contraction starts, when it ends, and how strong it is, than external contraction monitoring does. Of course, women are also good at reporting these sensations in labour. However, if an epidural is in place the sensation from contractions diminishes and the woman may not feel them anymore. Maternity professionals can feel contractions by placing a hand on the woman's uterus. Feeling for contractions, and the use of an external contraction sensor, is less accurate in heavier women, so intrauterine pressure catheters are sometimes recommended for this group of women (Frolova et al., 2021).

Three randomised controlled trials have compared external with internal contraction monitoring, all in groups of women where an infusion of the hormone oxytocin was being used to make contractions stronger (Bakkar et al., 2010; Chua et al., 1990; Hautakangas et al., 2020).

None of the trials showed significant differences in caesarean section or instrumental birth rates, in outcomes for the baby, or how long the labour was.

There has been no research comparing external with internal contraction monitoring for women who were not using an oxytocin infusion during their labour.

Telemetry or "wireless" CTG monitoring

The use of telemetry (wireless) CTG monitoring systems is increasingly common. There is a belief that telemetry systems support women's mobility in labour, can reduce their experience of labour pain, and the increased mobility might reduce the rise in caesarean section rates seen in the CTG monitoring research. *There have been no randomised controlled trials to know whether using telemetry rather than "wired" CTG monitoring has a substantial impact on these outcomes, or on outcomes for the baby.* There is very little research of any type that has explored telemetry CTG monitoring systems.

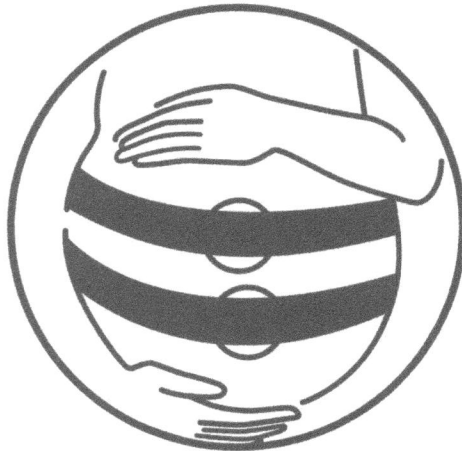

Telemetry or "wireless" CTG monitoring

One research team has studied women's experiences of using telemetry CTG monitoring (Watson et al., 2022). Women described better mobility with telemetry than with wired CTG monitoring, and as a consequence they felt more in control and less vulnerable. They appreciated being able to use the bathroom independently and the privacy of being able to shut the door while doing so, knowing this would not interfere with the CTG recording.

Watson also gathered information about the outcomes of women's labours when telemetry was and was not used. Women who had telemetry rather than "wired" CTG monitoring were more likely to give birth by caesarean section (22% vs 14%), less likely to use an epidural during labour (39% vs 46%), and more likely to give birth with a tear or episiotomy (26% vs 16%). It is important to note this study was not designed to show whether these outcomes were statistically different or not.

Telemetry systems are yet another example of a fetal monitoring technology that has been widely introduced with almost no research to establish whether it is a good idea or not.

"Beltless" CTG monitoring

Non-invasive fetal ECG monitoring, also known as "beltless" CTG monitoring, is new and not widely available. Like telemetry systems, non-invasive fetal ECG monitoring is "wireless" as there is no physical connection with the CTG machine. Non-invasive fetal ECG systems are "beltless" as the sensors are held in place with a sticky adhesive rather than with elastic belts. There is not a lot of research about these new monitoring systems as yet, and none of what has been done was designed to study whether this approach to CTG monitoring produced better outcomes for babies or women than any other approach to fetal heart rate monitoring.

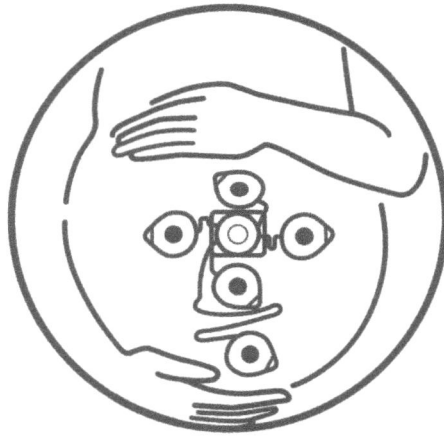

Non-invasive fetal ECG or "beltless" monitoring

In Australia, researchers have interviewed midwives in a hospital where a new "beltless" CTG monitoring system was being trialled (Fox, D. et al., 2022). They have also interviewed women who used the "beltless" system for their labour (Coddington et al., 2023). Women and midwives reported improved freedom of movement and comfort compared to "wired" CTG monitoring, but the system was not free of the need for midwives to "poke and prod" to maintain the CTG output.

While telemetry and "beltless" approaches seem to offer some additional comfort for women, they are both still forms of CTG monitoring. There is no reason to believe that either approach will produce different outcomes for babies than has been seen in randomised controlled trials for "wired" CTG systems.

Whether women's improved freedom of movement with "beltless" monitoring translates into more vaginal births, and fewer caesareans and instrumental births is unknown at present.

Fetal blood sampling

A Cochrane review has summarised reseach about whether fetal blood sampling can improve outcomes or not (East et al., 2015). They found two trials, both comparing pH measurement with lactate measurement (with no significant differences in outcomes for women or babies between the two options), and no research comparing any form of fetal blood sampling with none.

East later worked with a different team of researchers to compare CTG monitoring without a backup test, with CTG monitoring and the use of fetal blood sampling to measure lactate levels (East et al., 2021). They were not able to recruit the number of women they had planned to include in the trial. This prevented them from showing whether there was a difference in the caesarean section rate, or not, when fetal blood sampling was used in addition to the CTG. The only difference in outcomes for babies was a higher rate of low Apgar scores at five minutes of age among the group who were allocated to fetal blood sampling when the CTG was abnormal. This might be a sign that fetal lactate results generated false reassurance, so intervention was delayed when the fetal heart rate pattern was abnormal.

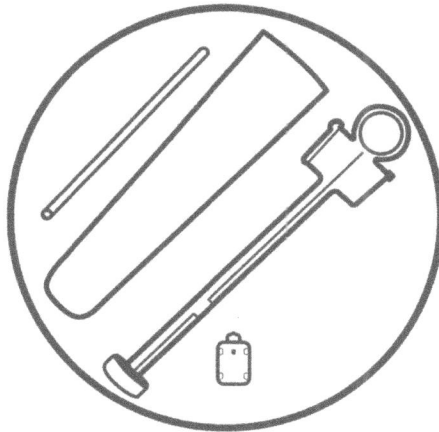

Equipment used for fetal blood sampling

One study looked at the ability of fetal blood sampling with pH testing to predict whether the baby would have a poor outcome after birth (Al Wattar et al., 2019). They found scalp pH results were not good at predicting outcomes. This could be because the theory that high levels of acid relate to low levels of oxygen may not be true after all.

Having the test done can be uncomfortable. A study from Sweden asked women to rate their pain after the procedure (Liljeström et al., 2014). Women using epidural analgesia rated the pain as three out of ten and those not using epidural analgesia rated it as seven out of ten. When the procedure took longer or was described as difficult by the obstetrician performing the test, pain scores were higher.

It seems logical to think that fetal blood sampling can avoid the overuse of caesarean section when CTG monitoring is in use by better selecting which babies really do have low oxygen levels and which do not. However, there is not enough evidence to know whether fetal blood sampling really can reduce the use of caesarean section.

Fetal scalp stimulation

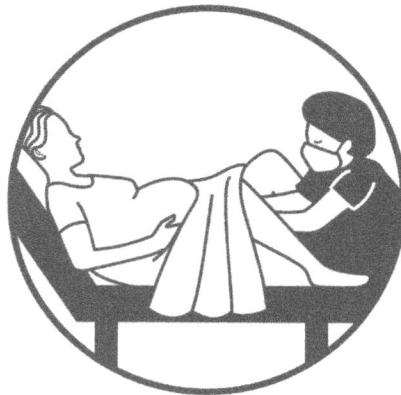

A health professional performing a vaginal examination to stimulate the fetal scalp

An approach often considered as an alternative to fetal blood sampling is fetal scalp stimulation. Fetal scalp stimulation is the practice of pinching or rubbing the fetal head through the open cervix using a finger or two. The theory is that any fetus who responds to such stimulation with a positive change in its heart rate pattern must have normal oxygen levels. Fetal scalp stimulation has been used when the CTG is abnormal to help decide whether to continue with labour or to end it sooner by caesarean section or instrumental birth.

Two recent randomised controlled trials have looked to see whether fetal stimulation might either improve outcomes for babies or reduce the use of caesarean section when the CTG was abnormal (Tahmina et al., 2022; Yambasu et al., 2025). The earlier study (Tahmina et al., 2022) compared fetal scalp stimulation with not using any backup test, while the most recent study (Yambasu, et al., 2025) compared it with fetal blood sampling. In both studies, the women in the group where fetal stimulation was used had the same caesarean section rate as the group of women where fetal stimulation was not used or fetal blood sampling was used instead. There were also no differences in outcomes for the babies in these two trials.

> At present, fetal scalp stimulation doesn't have sufficient research behind it to be clear about whether it is useful or not.

STAN

STAN is intended to provide additional information when the fetal heart rate pattern seen with CTG monitoring is not normal (you'll find a description of what STAN is back in chapter two). This extra information is used to help decide whether intervening in a woman's labour is likely to be a good idea or not. If STAN worked well, you would expect that women who were monitored by STAN in addition to the CTG would be less likely to give birth by caesarean section or instrumental birth than women monitored only with a CTG. It would be even better if adding STAN to the CTG meant that fewer babies would be born with high levels of acid, signs of brain injury (like seizures or hypoxic ischaemic encephalopathy), or die soon after birth.

In 2024, Blix and colleagues summarised what was known from nine randomised controlled trials, with 28,729 women, where STAN use alongside CTG monitoring was compared with CTG monitoring alone. They found no differences between the two groups for the use of caesarean section, instrumental birth, death of the baby, Apgar scores, encephalopathy, admission to the neonatal unit, or having a high level of acid in the umbilical cord blood at birth.

Norway has made widespread use of STAN. Blix and colleagues (2022) examined the real-world impact of the introduction of STAN systems on maternal and perinatal outcomes in this country. While the rate of stillbirth and neonatal death had fallen during the period 1985 to 2014 when the data for the study was collected, subsequent analysis showed that this was not related to the use of STAN technology. Similarly, while caesarean section and instrumental birth rates rose over time, this was also unrelated to the introduction of STAN systems.

Current research does not show that using STAN in addition to CTG monitoring improves outcomes for women or their babies.

Central fetal monitoring

Original CTG monitors generated a graph on paper. To read the CTG trace, professionals had to go to the birth room, or someone would tear the paper off the machine and bring the trace to them. As computer technology has advanced, it has become possible to collect data about the fetal heart rate and the woman's uterine contractions as digital data. This means the CTG trace can be generated as an image on a computer screen and stored as digital data.

Digitisation also means the CTG trace can be viewed in locations other than the birth room, in real time, so maternity professionals no longer need to enter the birth room if they want to see the CTG trace. Central fetal monitoring systems gather data from all the CTG machines in use and display this data on a screen in a location that is central within the birthing service – hence the name.

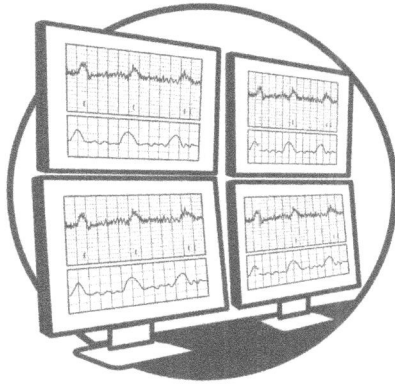

A bank of monitors showing multiple CTG recordings

Central fetal monitoring systems were designed with the goal of improving outcomes for babies. It is sometimes argued that being able to view the CTG without entering a woman's birth room avoids disruptions to her care and privacy. It is easier for there to be oversight over each CTG by many people, ideally senior obstetric, midwifery or nursing staff with significant expertise in interpreting and managing fetal heart rate patterns. The hope is that someone might recognise worrying fetal heart rate patterns that the midwife in the room has not noticed. Central fetal monitoring systems also make it possible for the woman to be left alone in the birth room during her labour while still having someone watch the CTGs. It is believed that these design features mean central fetal monitoring should improve care during labour and lead to better outcomes. These beliefs have led to the widespread introduction of central fetal monitoring systems in high-income countries.

Central fetal monitoring sounds like a great option!

However, there has never been a randomised controlled trial comparing "standard" CTG monitoring with central fetal monitoring to assess whether these beliefs about central fetal monitoring are true. Three studies have looked at what happened in hospitals where central monitoring was in use and was then turned off because of faults with the system (Brown et al., 2016; Weiss et al., 1997; Withiam-Leitch et al., 2006). No differences in any of the measured outcomes for the baby were seen between the period when central fetal monitoring was in use and when it was not. One of the hospitals documented a higher caesarean section rate when central monitoring was in use (Weiss et al., 1997), but this was not the case at the other two places.

In one of the studies (Brown et al., 2016), maternity professionals said they spent less time providing face-to-face care for birthing women when central monitoring was used. Choosing to leave the woman alone in the birth room was also described in research about central fetal monitoring from Iceland (Gottfreðsdottir et al., 2025). This has the potential to be less safe, as professionals might not notice early signs of a problem occurring if they are not in the room. There's also no guarantee that someone will notice a problem out at the central monitoring area. As one of the midwives I interviewed in my own research about central fetal monitoring said (Small et al., 2022, p. 198):

> You kind of assume that somebody's watching the CTG. So that you would kind of assume that if the trace is starting to go bad then you do hope that somebody's going to come down and help. But you can't guarantee anybody's looking at your trace and you can't guarantee someone's actually going to come down and help.

Some maternity units ensure there is a designated person whose role is to watch the central monitoring feed and ensure that appropriate responses are taken (Reavis, 2011), but this doesn't happen everywhere.

Central fetal monitoring systems and safety

While I hadn't intended to look at safety when planning my research on central fetal monitoring, it became clear that introducing the central monitoring system had changed the way maternity professionals behaved in ways that might potentially impact on safety. My colleagues and I wrote about this in a paper called "I'm not doing what I should be doing as a midwife" (Small et al., 2022). Some of the things we discussed were how:

✧ Maternity professionals made decisions about women's care at the central monitoring station without having all relevant information to help make those decisions and without involving the woman or her midwife.

✧ Midwives' work with birthing women was interrupted by other maternity professionals coming to the birth room in response to what were seen to be abnormal changes in the CTG when this was not appropriate (for example when the baby was being born). Sometimes this was accompanied by disrespectful behaviour by the professional entering the room. The midwife was often busy working to address the issue with the abnormal heart rate pattern and had to stop what they were doing to talk to the person who had come to the room.

✧ Midwives described a sense of anxiety about being constantly watched and thinking that someone was about to come into the birth room. This undermined midwives' confidence.

✧ Midwives spoke of their concerns that birthing women were frightened when people came into their room when they weren't expecting it.

✧ Midwives felt pressure to generate a "perfect" CTG recording that could be interpreted by an observer outside the room. They gave examples of limiting women's movements and coercing women to have a fetal spiral electrode placed to make the CTG look better. When the CTG was abnormal, midwives might rush the woman to push the baby out before people could come to the room. None of these things were being done because there was a problem for the baby, but to avoid people coming into the room.

✧ To try to keep people from coming to the birth room, midwives would write extra notes in the computer system. These were visible on the CTG at the central monitoring system. This communicated to the outside person that the midwife was aware that the CTG pattern was abnormal and was responding appropriately. While this meant better quality documentation, it drew midwives away from caring for the woman. The midwife quoted in the title of our paper said (p.188):

> I find I'm spending a lot of my time standing at [the computer]. I'm not talking to the woman, I'm not being 'with woman', and I'm not doing what I should be doing as a midwife.

These behaviours didn't happen every time a woman was being monitored by a CTG, but they were happening some of the time, and that's enough cause for concern. Each of the changes in behaviour I saw had the potential to make care less safe for women and their babies. Because we hadn't set out at the start to do a study about safety, I didn't collect data about things like changes in the caesarean section rate or whether more babies were admitted to the special care nursery, so I can't comment on these.

> It is vital that central fetal monitoring systems be properly assessed. We really should know whether they do achieve the improvements that have been promised before we continue to invest large amounts of money installing them.

It is of great concern to me that recent recommendations for changes to maternity care in the UK include the introduction of central fetal monitoring in all maternity services (Ockendon, 2022). There are no research findings to support this significant and expensive change.

Computer interpretation of the CTG

Collecting CTG information as digital data also made it possible to develop software that can interpret the CTG (Fergus et al., 2017). One of the arguments about why poor outcomes continue to occur with CTG monitoring relates to the maternity professional not recognising when the fetal heart rate pattern is significantly abnormal. Computer interpretation of the CTG is designed to address this by having standardised systems that are never tired, hungry, busy, or distracted, and consistently detect the same pattern as abnormal each time it appears. The theory is that professionals will be triggered to respond appropriately when the colour changes or the alarm goes off, and therefore outcomes will be better.

There have been several randomised controlled trials where computer interpretation has been compared to interpretation by maternity professionals alone. A team of researchers recently pulled all the research together (Tsipoura et al., 2023). They found five trials. There were no differences in caesarean or instrumental birth rates in the five trials.

The research they reported on showed no differences in any of the measured outcomes for the fetus or baby, with the exception of one study. That study (Nunes et al., 2017) found that computer interpretation was associated with a lower rate of babies having high levels of acid in the umbilical cord blood at birth, but no differences in rates of death, hypoxic ischaemic encephalopathy, or admission to the neonatal unit. I'm not convinced that we should pay much attention to the blood test results. If blood was not tested, no one would even have known there was an issue as it didn't make a difference to the sorts of outcomes that woman and families really want to know about.

> At this point in time, computer interpretation doesn't seem to lead to better outcomes that really count.

I'll talk more about these systems in the final chapter (looking at the future of fetal monitoring), as there is still a lot of development work going on to try to make computer interpretation systems work better.

Summary

Previous chapters explored evidence about whether CTG monitoring offered advantages over intermittent auscultation, or increased the chance of harm. This chapter looked at other things that have been added to, or done as part of, CTG monitoring with the aim of making it work better. So far, *none of the extra bits added to CTG monitoring appear to make it work any better at preventing poor outcomes for babies.* Some of the extra bits might push up the use of caesarean section and instrumental birth, and some could be making the way care is provided less safe and less comfortable.

It is important to note that when any of these options has been assessed in research, they are usually assessed one at a time. That's not what happens in practice though. A woman might find that central fetal monitoring with computer interpretation is used where she plans to give birth, and her maternity care provider recommends a fetal spiral electrode attached to a telemetry connection. How each of these interacts with one another is unknown. Perhaps having a multi-pronged approach like this gathers up any small benefit from each and magnifies it. It may also be possible that what happens is that all the downsides are multiplied together.

We really do need more research on these "extra bits". In an ideal world, there would be a pause on their use outside of research projects until we can better understand the impact of their use. Knowing in advance whether any of these options might be used where you plan to give birth helps you make decisions aimed at staying in control of your birth.

CHAPTER 7

It's your decision

The decision about which fetal heart rate monitoring method to use is a big decision, mostly because what is common in practice is not backed up by evidence of a better outcome. Women who decide to use an evidence-based fetal monitoring approach – like intermittent auscultation – can encounter significant pressure to conform to what the maternity service wants them to use. In this chapter you will find my suggestions about questions to ask to help you make your decision. You will also find tips on how to communicate your decision effectively.

Let's pause and refresh

Let me summarise where we are up to before we move forward. There is a small chance that low oxygen levels during labour can lead to death or permanent injury to the fetus or baby. CTG monitoring during labour was introduced in the hope it would reduce the chance of death or permanent injury better than the existing approach known as intermittent auscultation. CTG monitoring was rapidly introduced in the 1960s and became routine in maternity services in most high-income countries. Many maternity professionals have strongly held beliefs that CTG monitoring is a better option than using no heart rate monitoring, or using intermittent auscultation.

However, when we look at the research, this belief looks like nonsense. There is no strong evidence showing that using CTG monitoring in labour was better than intermittent auscultation for preventing death or permanent brain injury for the fetus / baby. This was true whether women had risk factors for poor outcomes or not. There was a small reduction in the chance that a baby would develop seizures soon after birth when CTG monitoring was used rather than intermittent auscultation, but this didn't translate to lower rates of brain injury as the child grew older. The reduction in seizures seemed to be mostly for women whose labour was being induced or sped up with an oxytocin infusion. The way oxytocin is used today is different so this may, or may not, apply any more.

Rates of caesarean section and instrumental birth were higher when CTG monitoring was used rather than with intermittent auscultation. Rates of vaginal birth were lower. There is no convincing evidence that adding additional technology (like central fetal monitoring or computer interpretation) to the CTG made it work better for the fetus / baby or made CTG use safer for the woman. We have no research to help us know whether using no fetal heart rate monitoring is better or worse than using either CTG monitoring or intermittent auscultation for women or for babies.

Despite what is known in research, professional guidelines in all high-income countries recommend CTG use in labour for women who are considered to be at increased risk for a poor outcome. When you then arrive in a maternity service in labour, particularly if you have something that appears on a list of risk factors, what is likely to happen? You might be advised to have CTG monitoring – and you might find that significant pressure is applied to get you to go along with this.

Etta's experience of decision-making

Etta's labour was induced. Her obstetrician advised her that the slightly higher risk that came from being over the age of 35 for her first birth could be reduced if she were induced just before her due date. Her obstetrician didn't mention anything about different ways to monitor her baby in labour when they spoke about what would happen with the induction.

Etta arrived at the hospital on the day of her induction. The midwife had laid out two straps on the hospital bed and asked Etta to hop up while her partner moved her bags into the room. Without further discussion, the midwife lifted Etta's shirt and wrapped the straps around her belly, securing the two sensors for the CTG in place. She then turned the CTG machine on and silently typed some information onto the screen. Eventually she turned the screen around, and pointed to the top line, saying "This is your baby's heart rate and he looks happy. The bottom line will show your contractions once they get started. I'll leave you here for a bit and will be back when your obstetrician comes to start your induction."

When Etta's obstetrician arrived, she ruptured her membranes. During the examination she said "I'm attaching a monitor clip to your baby. It'll save us having to do it later." CTG monitoring was used through the full duration of Etta's induced labour.

Novah's experience of decision-making

At 37 weeks, Novah and her midwife met to discuss her birth plans. She had read through the information her midwife had provided her and felt like she had a good understanding of the different options and the pros and cons of each. Her written birth plan said that she wanted to use intermittent auscultation and if there was a clinical concern then she would agree to the use of CTG monitoring.

About 2 hours after she arrived at the hospital in labour, Novah's midwife said that she was going to put the CTG on as she thought the heart rate was higher than when she last listened. Novah agreed. Her midwife left the room soon after and was gone for what seemed like a long time. Novah wanted to use the toilet, so she removed the straps and headed to the bathroom.

Suddenly two people she had not met before came into the bathroom while she was still on the toilet, working through a particularly strong contraction. One took her by the arm and said "we need to get you back to the bed and get the monitor back on right away!" Novah's partner stepped in and asked what was going on. They explained that they had been watching Novah's CTG trace at the central monitoring station. When they saw the heart rate suddenly disappear they were worried there was something wrong. Novah felt that she had no choice other than to agree to have the CTG put back on. Even though the fetal heart rate pattern remained normal for the rest of her labour, none of the people involved in her care gave her the option of using intermittent auscultation instead.

Who is making the decision about fetal monitoring?

Both these situations illustrate some aspect of fetal monitoring being used without the woman's explicit consent. Etta was never given information nor an opportunity to take part in making decisions about CTG and fetal spiral electrode use. She simply assumed she had no choice. Novah was informed and, at least initially, was involved in making decisions. Once in labour however, she found herself in a vulnerable position and without the support of the maternity professionals caring for her to use her preferred option for fetal monitoring. Are experiences like Etta's and Novah's rare, or commonplace?

Over the past 20 years, several researchers in a variety of different countries have explored the question of who the decision-maker is when it comes to fetal monitoring methods. I'm going to take you through this research, so you understand why may find yourself being pressured into using a particular approach to fetal monitoring. The research will also provide some ideas about what to watch out for to make sure you aren't being driven up a one-way road that is hard to back out of.

In England in 2008, researchers asked women whether they were given enough information to make a choice about how to monitor the baby's heartbeat in labour (Hindley et al., 2008). Only 40% of women answered yes. In Australia in 2012, nine percent of women reported having been given both information about fetal monitoring options in labour and a choice about what to use (Thompson & Miller, 2014). Findings from a later Australian study (Miller et al., 2022), showed that using CTG monitoring without the women's consent was less common in midwifery-led care than in medical-led care. In the USA, 24% of women felt pressured to use CTG monitoring, and only 26% recalled being asked what they wanted to do for fetal monitoring (Logan et al., 2022). Black and Indigenous women were more likely to experience fetal monitoring care they didn't consent to in this study, as were women who had medical-led rather than midwifery-led care.

The situation in Australia doesn't appear to have improved all that much over time, with a study in 2024 (Levett et al.) finding that only 35% of women were asked for consent for the type of fetal heart rate monitoring that was used during their labour, with four in every five women saying they were not given enough information about their options. Women who experienced intermittent auscultation were more likely to say they were given enough information about that choice (68%), than women who experienced "wired" CTG use (47%), or "wireless" CTG use (41%). An appallingly low proportion of women who had experienced the use of a fetal spiral electrode, only three percent, said they were given enough information about that option.

The only research I can find that appears to suggest anything different comes from Ireland (McMahon et al., 2019). I think the reason for this difference lies in the specific question asked, which was: did the staff caring for you explain your baby's heart rate monitoring to you? All women in this study answered yes to this question. There is no way of knowing what these explanations involved and whether they included accurate information and asked women what they wanted to do. I suspect a large proportion of women in this study will have had communication along the lines of – "because of your risk factors, you are going to need to have CTG monitoring". While this does count as an explanation, it is clearly inadequate.

How midwives have conversations about fetal monitoring

Why do I suspect that the way information was communicated in this Irish study was inadequate? Because there is a body of research that has looked at the kinds of conversations midwives have with women about fetal heart rate monitoring options for labour. Interestingly, researchers have never asked obstetricians the same questions, so we don't know for sure whether the same things are true for them or not.

In 2005, midwifery researchers Hindley and Thomson asked midwives in England if they knew what informed choice was. This is the concept that people should be offered both information and a choice to decide for themselves on all aspects of their healthcare. All the midwives they interviewed knew what informed choice was and agreed it was important. When the researchers then asked follow-up questions about how they approached conversations with women about fetal monitoring in labour, the message was very different, as illustrated by this quote from one of the midwives:

> Sometimes it's just biased information isn't it? You give them the information you want to give them, that you want them to have. (Paula, p. 310)

Norwegian midwives (Blix & Öhlund, 2007) said much the same thing:

> I can get the woman to do exactly what I want. Nearly always. If I am a bit... a bit, sort of, clever and sympathetic, I can get her exactly where I want her. ... I choose my words in a way so that she will not protest, it is the way I am asking her. I can also ask in a way that gives her the opportunity to choose, or make her say no. It depends on my way of asking. (Midwife 5, p. 55)

I saw something similar in my own research in Australia (Small et al., 2023), with one of the midwives I interviewed saying:

> I think the conversation about the CTG is carefully worded, so that nobody can come back and think you influenced her decision, especially if you are influencing her decision against hospital policy. I would never say outright, well the CTG is absolutely your choice, and you don't have to have it if you don't want to. You just go, well everything in your labour is absolutely your decision. Then leave it to her. (p. 284)

At this hospital, policy said that all women with one or more things on a long list of risk factors *must* have CTG monitoring. What you can see going on for this midwife is the recognition that making women aware that the decision about CTG monitoring is theirs to make will put the midwife's practice at odds with their responsibilities as an employee of that hospital. But the eventual solution of being deliberately vague and leaving it up to the woman to fill in the blanks is inadequate. Doing so means that many women never know they have a choice and they would not be offered information to support them when making that decision.

In this case, policy was clearly driving the midwife's actions, and this has been confirmed as one of the main reasons professionals communicate this way in other research (Chuey et al., 2020; Small et al., 2023). Other explanations for midwives' communication styles are the fear of being sued or reported to a professional body, or of being in conflict with their colleagues (Chuey et al., 2020; Ford et al., 2022).

> Maternity professionals who work in hospitals face strong pressures to use CTG monitoring, and as a result, they don't always provide accurate information or make it clear to women that this is the woman's decision to make.

It is your decision

This is the most important thing I want you to take from this book. Every decision during your pregnancy, labour, birth, and afterwards is for YOU to make. This includes all the decisions about fetal heart rate monitoring too. This is true whether you are considered high risk or not. It is true wherever you plan to give birth, and with whatever maternity professional you choose (or if you choose not to have any). It remains true even when someone tells you that you don't have a choice and that CTG monitoring is mandatory.

So how do you go about making these decisions?

Some women find it easier to make decisions than others for all sorts of reasons. Some have their own tried-and-tested processes to help them make decisions. Other women have had fewer opportunities to make their own decisions and be responsible for them. There are potentially a lot of decisions to make during pregnancy, birth, and parenting. If you haven't had many opportunities to do so before, pregnancy can give you the chance to develop your decision-making skills.

Decision making can be hard work and you don't have to do it on your own. You might even decide to let someone else make some, or all, of these decisions for you. That's a decision too. Delegating decision making to someone else works best when the person making the decisions for you knows you well, will share in the consequences of that decision, and you trust them to look after your best interests. Some people choose to let their maternity professional make the decisions. While this can seem like a good idea, be aware there is evidence that because of the way institutions work, maternity professionals often make decisions that fit the routines of their place of work, or that benefit their employer or themselves, rather than what is best for you (Newnham & Kirkham, 2019; Newnham et al., 2017).

It is important to be aware there is no risk screening process, no blood test or ultrasound, no individual profession or professional, no hospital or clinic, and no treatment plan that can guarantee a perfect outcome for every woman and every baby, every time. Even for approaches that really do reduce the chance of bad things happening, none remove that possibility completely. Some approaches to care might reduce the chance of a poor outcome for the baby but at the same time increase the chance of a poor outcome for the woman. How people balance these chances against each other is different for each person.

Recognise when you have a decision to make

You've seen the research showing that maternity professionals won't always make it clear when there is a decision being made about fetal heart rate monitoring. It is useful to be alert to the sorts of things maternity professionals might say that give you a clue about when a decision is being made, and you are not the one doing the deciding. Look out for things like:

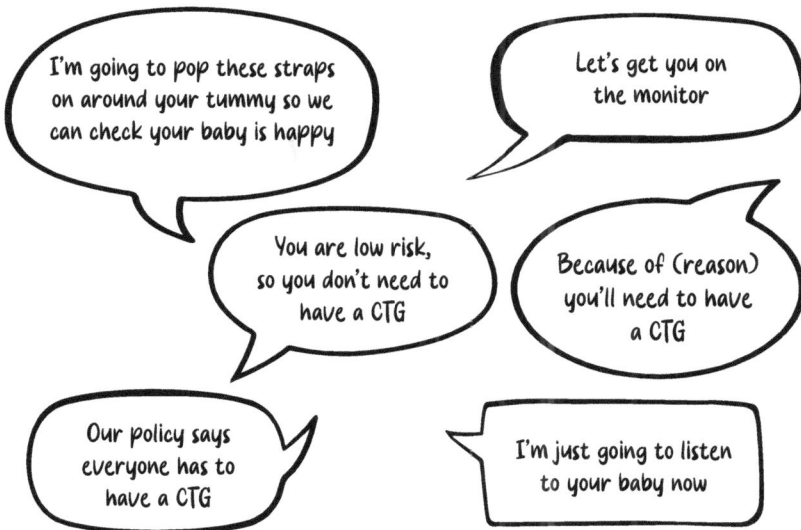

I'm going to pop these straps on around your tummy so we can check your baby is happy

Let's get you on the monitor

You are low risk, so you don't need to have a CTG

Because of (reason) you'll need to have a CTG

Our policy says everyone has to have a CTG

I'm just going to listen to your baby now

When you hear things like this, recognise that this is a time when someone, other than you, is deciding about the type of fetal heart rate monitoring that you will use.

If you find yourself in a situation where something like this is happening, it can be useful to slow the maternity professional down by asking a question or two. Your support partner can also step in here and ask these questions so you can focus on your labour. Ask something like "Can you explain why you are advising this, and what the pros and cons are, so I can decide whether this is what I want?". Even if you already know the pros and cons, this is a useful statement. A statement like this reminds the maternity professional that *you* are the decision-maker, and that they have a professional responsibility to provide you with information and then support your decision. If you are already clear about what you want to do, you could say "Thanks, for your suggestion. I have decided that I will (use intermittent auscultation, have CTG monitoring – whatever your decision is)."

Questions to ask yourself

Being clear in your own mind about what you want is an important step in making and expressing your decisions. With that in mind, here are some questions to ponder and to discuss with the people closest to you, if you want to.

1. *What are your personal risk factors?* Do you have any health conditions, previous pregnancy and birth experiences, or a history of previous pregnancy and birth experiences among family members that might mean a higher chance of a poor outcome for you and / or your baby? Maternity professionals and women can interpret the significance of these factors in different ways. Be clear about any risks in your own mind before you have a conversation about risk with your maternity professional. Balance these out against any protective factors that reduce the chance of a poor outcome.

2. *Can you change any of your risk factors?* Many risk factors (how old you are, whether you have given birth before) you can't do anything about, but there are some that you can change. Stopping smoking during pregnancy is an example of a risk factor you can change.

3. *Would more tests be useful to you or not?* Further tests might provide more information about risks. For instance, having an ultrasound scan showing your baby is of normal size and the blood flow through the placenta is normal, suggests a lower risk of poor outcomes. However, there is a chance that more testing might show your risk is higher than you thought. Before choosing further testing, make sure you ask whether there is clear evidence that knowing the results of the test can change the chance you will have a poor outcome. Not all the tests we use in maternity care have evidence of benefit, so you can be left in the uncomfortable position of knowing there is a higher risk but not being able to change that. More tests also create the potential for more things to be added to your "risk list" and that can mean more pushback from maternity professionals when you ask for your decisions to be respected.

4. *What matters to you?* Do you want to give birth in a birth centre, a hospital, at home, or somewhere else? Is vaginal birth really important to you? Do you plan to be induced or wait for labour to start? Do you want to remain mobile and upright during labour and birth or not? Are you planning to use water (shower / bath / birth pool) during your labour, and do you want to give birth in water? What plans do you have for coping with the physical sensations of your labour? Many of these plans will overlap with approaches to fetal heart rate monitoring in labour, as some monitoring approaches make it easier to be mobile and get into a birth pool for example.

5. *What are you fearful about?* Fear often drives decision making. This isn't necessarily wrong, but when fear takes over it can be hard to use the rational parts of our brain and we can make decisions that we later regret. Knowledge can help to overcome fear. For example, a woman might be fearful of stillbirth in labour because it happened to a work colleague. Knowing how uncommon stillbirth is might help to reduce that fear so it becomes easier to manage. Sometimes people have a persistent fear that doesn't shift with extra knowledge. Good counselling might help and provides

useful skills to apply to other fearful situations in life. As you make decisions, ask yourself am I choosing this because I am fearful? Would I make the same decision if I didn't have this fear?

6. *What do or don't I have on my side?* Each of us have limits on our time, energy, and money. Do you have access to "free" maternity care? Do you have health insurance and if so, what does it cover? What maternity services are available in your local area and what does each service offer? Sometimes in life there is a distinction between the best option, and the option that is realistic given the actual circumstances of your life. Knowing in advance what your limits are can help. Sometimes you can change your situation (like purchasing different insurance, or changing your care provider), depending on how much time you have before you expect to be giving birth.

Being clear in your own mind about what you want, what you don't want, why, and what you can and can't access provide a firm base from which to make your own decisions.

Finding a maternity professional to work with

I really, very strongly, recommend that you find and work with one main maternity professional through your pregnancy, birth, and the first weeks after birth. Ideally that should be a midwife. Having one person as your go-to care provider is called continuity of carer. Continuity of carer doesn't mean that you can't add in care from someone else. If you need to see someone with specific expertise about a particular issue, that should happen, while you continue to have your continuity provider involved in your care.

Why is continuity of carer important? Women who have continuity of carer are more likely to be given information to help them make decisions, be asked what their decision is, and to be supported in making that decision happen (Logan et al., 2022; Miller et al., 2022). There is sound evidence that pregnant women who have continuity of carer, where that carer is a midwife, have better outcomes (Sandall et al., 2024).

Women who received midwifery continuity of carer were less likely to give birth by caesarean section, forceps or vacuum, experience an episiotomy, with no differences in rates of stillbirth or death of the baby after birth, or the rate of admission to the neonatal nursery. Women described their care more favourably and there were cost savings for healthcare systems.

Midwifery continuity of carer can look very different in different parts of the world. Do some research about what is available in your local area. You may be able to access midwifery care at no cost through a government funded maternity hospital or community-based service (they are sometimes called midwifery group practices). In some places, you will find this style of care on offer in birth centres. You might choose a midwife working in their own private practice and pay them for your care, if you can afford this option. Some midwives in private practice only provide care for women planning to birth at home, while others can be your carer for your birth in a birth centre or a hospital.

Midwifery continuity of carer is not universally available. If you can't access this, then the next best option is to have a stable relationship with one care giver – an obstetrician or (in some parts of the world) a general practitioner / family physician, or some other professional with expertise in maternity care. Ideally, this should be the same person who is going to provide you care when you are in labour and during the weeks after your birth. If you are already seeing a carer, ask them how likely it is that they will be the person who provides your care when you give birth and afterwards.

When you have an ongoing professional relationship with one maternity professional, there is time over the course of your pregnancy for each of you to get to know the other well, and to develop trust. There is time for information sharing, to think about your options, and to communicate what you want your care to look like. Having the same care provider for labour as during your pregnancy means you won't have to go back over the information again and justify your decisions to a new person who doesn't know you or the progress of your pregnancy in detail.

If your relationship with your current professional(s) isn't working well, consider changing your care provider.

Questions to ask your maternity professional

Whether you have a continuity relationship with one person or not, there are some questions about fetal heart rate monitoring in labour it is useful to ask the professional caring for you. Ideally, aim to have these conversations during your pregnancy, so you have time to think and decide. If you have a different care provider once you are in labour, you may need to run through some of these again. If you have a support person – such as your partner, a family member, friend, or doula – they might do this so you can focus on your labour. Your maternity professional might be proactive in discussing fetal heart rate monitoring with you, or they may not. Most guidelines for maternity professionals recommend that fetal heart rate monitoring in labour is discussed with every woman during her pregnancy, so if this hasn't happened yet, it is okay for you to ask to talk about it.

Here are my suggestions for things to ask, and for each one I explain why the answer to these questions is important.

1. *What are my risk factors? What are the things I am at higher risk of happening? Exactly what is the chance of that happening or is this something that we simply don't know?* While you have your own knowledge about your risks, your professionals' understanding of your risk factors will shape the care they want to provide to you. Being on the same page about risk can be helpful. You can also ask about any protective factors that reduce the chance of a problem happening.

2. *What are your policies (and / or those of the service where you plan to give birth) regarding fetal heart rate monitoring during labour? Is there flexibility in the policy?* Policies have a big impact

on what maternity professionals do. Even if your maternity professional is employed by you rather than a health service, and you are planning on giving birth outside a hospital, the policies of the hospital you might use if you decide to transfer there during labour, the professional standards of your chosen care provider, and the health department policies of the state or country you live in, still impact their practice. If you know what your maternity professional is expected to do in relation to fetal heart rate monitoring, then you will be in a good position to make sense of the recommendations they give to you.

3. *Can I have a copy of the policies about fetal heart rate monitoring that you use?* A maternity professional who is willing to share information is someone that is likely to work with you to help you achieve your goals for your birth. Well written policies will include references to up-to-date evidence that you might find useful if you want more information as you decide the best course of action.

4. *If I make a decision that is not recommended in this policy, what might the response be? Will my decision be supported?* It is far better to find out well ahead of time whether you can expect to be treated with respect and have your decisions supported, or whether you might be refused care or treated disrespectfully. If your professional indicates they will not respect your decisions, don't try to convince them, and hope they will change their mind. Find another professional who will listen to you (this might be a more senior midwife or obstetrician), or another maternity service if this is an option.

5. *What equipment is available for fetal heart rate monitoring?* Finding that waterproof telemetry (wireless) monitoring is not available, or there are no handheld Dopplers, or some other form of fetal monitoring you had planned to have, once you are already in labour at the location where you intend to give birth, is frustrating. It is usually too late to make different arrangements at that point. While you might have planned on using only one

approach to fetal heart rate monitoring, I would suggest that knowing about alternative options is also useful. You can't predict in advance what might unfold and having a plan B and C available to you could be useful and reassuring.

6. *What approaches to fetal heart rate monitoring do you have expertise with?* Not all maternity professionals have well developed skills with intermittent auscultation, particularly with devices that don't use Doppler technology. Professionals who work mostly outside of hospitals (providing home or birth centre care) may not have much experience with CTG monitoring. If your professional has limited expertise with a particular approach, ask what their backup plan would be if you decided to use that approach.

7. *If you have concerns about the fetal heart rate pattern, do you offer additional tests to help decide whether it is safe to continue my labour?* If you are using intermittent auscultation, will your professional advise you to change to CTG monitoring at the first suggestion of a problem, or continue using intermittent auscultation while they work out what is going on? If CTG monitoring with external sensors are in use, will they suggest a fetal spiral electrode? Fetal stimulation, fetal blood sampling for pH or lactate testing, or ST segment analysis (STAN) might be suggested to try to determine whether caesarean or instrumental birth is a better option than continuing with labour. As discussed in chapter six, these each have their own pros and cons so it is worth considering in advance what you might choose if one or other of these might be offered to you.

8. *Does this hospital have central fetal monitoring? Who can see my trace? Can my tracing be turned off if I don't want my information shared at the central monitoring area?* It has been my experience that central fetal monitoring systems are a bit like the floor covering in the birth room: once installed, people forget about it and don't go out of their way to let you know that it is there. If you are concerned about the impact central fetal monitoring might

have on your privacy, or on your chance of being advised to have a caesarean birth, it might be possible to have the CTG recording of your baby's heart rate not be displayed at the central monitoring station, or it might not.

9. *Does this hospital use computer interpretation of the CTG?* Like central fetal monitoring, computer interpretation systems tend to be invisible and not something maternity professionals think to mention in advance. You are unlikely to know that computer software is providing interpretation information about your CTG recording unless you specifically ask about it. If computer interpretation of the CTG is in use at the hospital where you plan to give birth, you won't be able to opt out of this if you use CTG monitoring. That may or may not impact on your decisions about having CTG monitoring.

Navigating your way to a decision

You now have more knowledge about what research says about different fetal heart rate monitoring options; knowledge about whether you have factors that change your chance of a problem arising during labour, your goals for your birth, and any practical limits you face; and knowledge about your maternity professional and any limitations they may face in supporting your decision. Now you can consider the potential benefits and possible harms for each fetal monitoring option, in relation to what you feel is right for you and your unborn baby, within the limits of what is available to you in your specific situation. And that's how you end up with your decision about what you plan to use for fetal monitoring for your labour.

I recommend having a "best case scenario" plan – assuming everything during your labour unfolds as you hoped it would – and to also have some extra plans up your sleeve for when unexpected things happen. If you develop a complication prior to or during your labour (like bleeding or pre-eclampsia) and the chance of a poor outcome goes up, what do you want to do under those circumstances? If your experience with your chosen monitoring approach is not as you expected, what would you like to try next? If the equipment you planned to use isn't available, what is the next best option? A good decision-making process leaves you space to adjust the plan as new information comes to light.

Some people prefer to write their plans down to help them think things through, some don't. Some people prefer to make decisions on their own, while others find it useful to talk through their ideas with another person. If you are feeling stuck, it is worthwhile remembering you have already made millions of decisions during your lifetime. It might be helpful if you can think back to other times when you had to make a big decision, one where you felt that decision turned out to have been a good one and reflect on the process you used. See if it might help you once again.

Communicating your decision

You have made up your mind. Now it is time to talk about telling your maternity professional what you want. Women sometimes end up in a position where it is easy for others to take charge as we have been socialised to be nice, to not rock the boat, to not get pushy. You might think it is easier to wait until your maternity professional brings up the issue of fetal monitoring, hoping that they will offer you exactly what you want. I would strongly recommend against that approach. "Going with the flow" can seem like the easiest way to negotiate maternity care. But when it comes to fetal monitoring in labour, the direction of that flow is towards a lack of choice, increasingly intense levels of surveillance, and more intervention. If that's not what you want, you need to be prepared to take action to go against the direction of the flow.

This is your body, your baby, and your birth, and you aren't going to give birth very often, or possibly ever again. So – commit to doing whatever you need to do to make your birth a positive experience.

> The key to getting what you want is to communicate what you have decided, not ask for permission.

Consider what will most likely happen if you say things like:

> If I want to have a vaginal birth after my previous caesarean section, do I need to have CTG monitoring?

> Am I allowed to have time off the CTG if I want to go in the shower?

These statements assume the person who has the authority to make this decision is the maternity professional, not you. These questions show the maternity professional that you believe you need their permission to do what you want in relation to fetal monitoring. Yet, this isn't the case. Anything a health professional wants to do to your body requires your permission, not the other way around. In response to these questions the maternity professional is likely to say yes, you need CTG monitoring, or no you can't come off the CTG, and if those were not what you wanted – you now find yourself in a pickle where you need to either "break the rules" or let go of the decision you made.

Instead of ending up in this situation, consider the impact of saying:

> I have decided I will start with intermittent auscultation, and I'll let you know if I change my mind as things change during my labour. I'd like you to note that in my records, so I don't have to explain again when I come to hospital.

Statements like this not only communicate your decision, but your awareness that you are the decision-maker.

It is important to be really clear in your communication that this is you telling them what you have decided, not you wanting to open up a discussion about your choices (unless you actually want to because you want more information). Think about this statement:

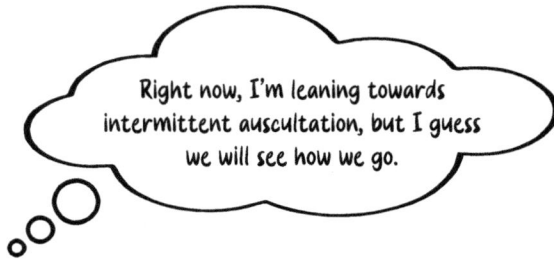

> Right now, I'm leaning towards intermittent auscultation, but I guess we will see how we go.

You might think this says the same thing as the previous statement, but it would be very easy for a maternity professional to interpret this as an opening for them to attempt to change your mind, either now, or once you are in labour.

Practice making confident statements about your plans for birth until you can do it comfortably. Stand in front of a mirror, or do it with another person, until you can say it without feeling weird. When you show you are clear about what you have decided, it makes it easier for maternity professionals to recognise your decision is a decision, not an invitation to talk you into doing what they want you to do instead.

What to do if you encounter resistance

I'd love to be able to promise you that if you do the things I have already suggested, then your maternity professional will respect your decision and support you by making it happen without fuss. There is a chance that they will push back and try to exert control to get you to do what they have decided you should have. Here are some statements you can try if this happens. Having your support person repeat the same statement, preceded by "She said-" can help too.

> That's not an option I am willing to consider at this point

> I would accept that option, but only if (reason). Right now I want...

> Thanks. My decision remains the same

> I want to transfer my care to someone who will respect my decision

> I SAID NO!

> I don't consent to that

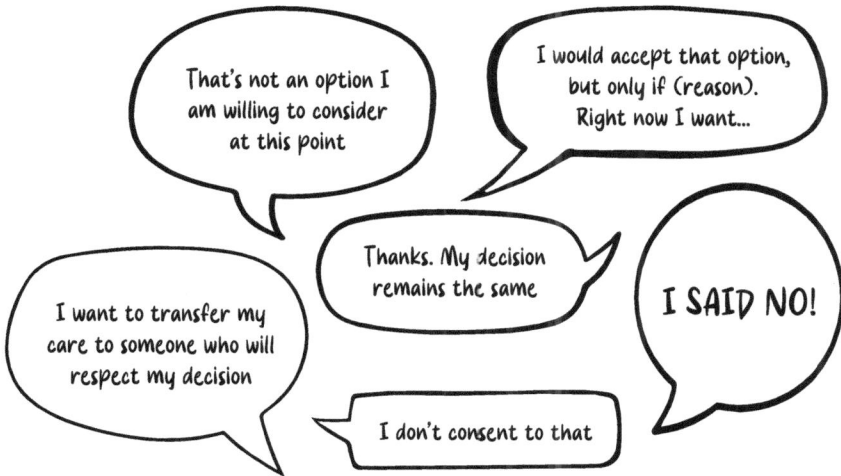

It is important to know what your rights are, in the healthcare system where you are receiving care. In some places, maternity professionals can not refuse to provide you with professional support if you decline one or more recommendations. In other places, they can do this. Do some online searching to find out what your situation is, so you know in advance whether you can demand a certain fetal monitoring approach without the risk of having care withdrawn.

Be mindful that there is one situation that is particularly tricky when it comes to standing your ground on your choice of fetal monitoring approach. And that is when you want your maternity professionals to perform or arrange an intervention for you where CTG monitoring is considered part of the package deal. Induction of labour and the use of an epidural for pain management are the two examples that come to mind for me. While you can insist that you will have intermittent auscultation, the professional might refuse to go ahead with the intervention if CTG monitoring is considered part of the deal. You will need to decide whether to go ahead with the intervention with CTG monitoring, or continue with intermittent auscultation and not have the intervention.

Two things that are not your job

First, *you don't need to explain to your maternity professional why you made your choice, or back your decisions up with evidence, if you don't want to.* From time to time, I have people approach me asking for evidence they can show to their maternity professional to get them to change their mind about what they are recommending. Educating your maternity professional about what the research says is not your job.

And second, it isn't your job to manage your maternity professional's emotional response to your decision. Women have often been raised to keep track of the emotional vibe of all the people around them and to behave in ways that maximise comfort levels for those people. When it to comes to communicating your fetal monitoring decision, the urge to not let down, or upset, your maternity professional when making a decision that is best for you but not what they want, is not at all helpful. If you find yourself stuck in a cycle of worry about telling them your decision, you may find it helpful to remind yourself that how they respond emotionally is out of your control and has nothing to do with you.

Your job is to decide. Their job is to respect your decision. Getting your maternity professional to change their recommendation or their emotional response to your decision is not your job, and it will almost certainly not work.

Yes, I know, and I'm sorry

You might be thinking, "this is really hard! Why do I need to be the one doing the deciding and the communicating? Shouldn't my maternity professional do this for me?" I get it. Making and communicating a decision about fetal monitoring should not be difficult. Yet it sometimes can be. If you experience this, know that this is a symptom of a maternity system that is not functioning well.

We should have a maternity system where professionals always respect and listen to women, provide recommendations based on evidence from well conducted research, and support women's decisions. Instead, we have a system where guideline recommendations about fetal monitoring don't match up with evidence and where it is easier for maternity professionals if they can get women to do what the guideline says.

Sometimes getting what you want from your maternity care happens by pure luck. At other times it is because you are strong, well educated, well supported, and you didn't give up until you got what was best for you. While it is awesome that some women can do that for themselves, it also bothers me. Women who don't speak English, can't read, are socially isolated, or have been traumatised in the past might be unable to stand up for themselves in this way. These women shouldn't get worse care than persistent, strong, educated, supported women, but they sometimes do. We know there are worse outcomes for disempowered and marginalised women from national reports on the outcomes of maternity care in all our high-income countries (like the most recent Saving Lives, Improving Mother's Care report from the UK, Felker et al., 2024).

I, like many others working in maternity research and education, continue to push for change so respectful, evidence-based approaches to care are the standard. If you want to contribute, there are organisations and social media-based groups that you can join to help push for a better maternity system.

Summary

The type of fetal heart rate monitoring used during your labour and birth is your decision. In this chapter I explored ways to help you decide what you want, and to communicate your decision to your maternity professional. Before we reach the end of the book, let's look to the future to see what new options for monitoring the fetus during labour might be just across the horizon.

CHAPTER 8

What does the future hold?

Technology development continues to provide new approaches for monitoring fetal wellbeing during labour. Some new technologies are starting to move from research into use in practice, so you might come across them. Others are a long way from being turned into reality but provide hope that we might have better solutions at some point. In this chapter, I will explore future horizons for fetal monitoring in labour and why I think that the best option will be something other than monitoring the fetal heart rate.

Making CTG monitoring more comfortable – "beltless" systems

I have already touched on these systems in chapter two. Externally worn CTG sensors are uncomfortable. Noninvasive fetal ECG (Ni-fECG) or "beltless" CTG monitoring records the fetal heart rate and uterine contractions reliably from external sensors that don't require the use of belts to hold them in place.

Researchers have started to evaluate "beltless" systems. So far, we have no research examining the impact these systems have on outcomes for the mother or baby compared to traditional CTG monitoring, or compared with intermittent auscultation. Given what we know about CTG monitoring – and knowing that these systems use the same data (heart rate and contractions) in the same way as other approaches to CTG monitoring – it seems unlikely they will lead to better outcomes for women and babies than "regular" CTG monitoring approaches.

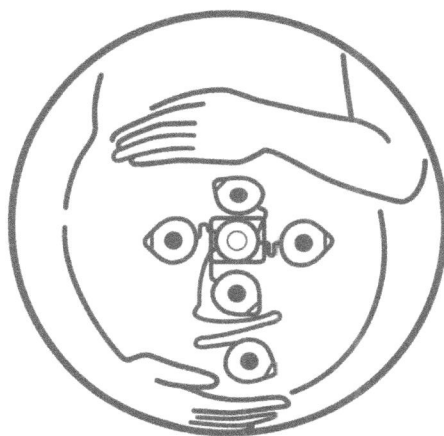

"Beltless" CTG monitoring

What we know from research so far is "beltless" systems provide more continuous information about the fetal heart rate than Doppler based CTG systems that are prone to having episodes where the fetal heart rate can't be detected or can be confused with the woman's heart rate (Cohen, et al., 2012; Hayes-Gill, et al., 2020). Doppler recording of the fetal heart rate is more challenging in women with a high body mass index. "Beltless" monitoring does a better job of recording the heart rate continuously for this group of women (Cohen, et al., 2014; Euliano, et al., 2017).

It is important to bear in mind that more reliable detection of the fetal heart rate in research doesn't translate to perfect recording, all the time in actual practice. A recent Australian study of 110 women (Fox, et al., 2021) reported the device they were using (Phillips Avalon Beltless Solution or PABS) was not able to be used at all by 27% of the women, and only 24% of women used "beltless" Ni-fECG through the full duration of labour. For some of these women, the decision to switch to a different monitor related to their intention to use water immersion.

The same Australian team interviewed midwives about their experience of using the "beltless" system in a small pilot study (Fox, D., et al., 2022). Midwives felt that the "beltless" system had a positive impact on women's mobility and comfort in labour. When the system worked well, it required less midwifery time to maintain an interpretable trace, freeing midwives up to be "with woman" rather than "with machine". As one midwife said:

> I feel like you can just kind of be there with them and talk then through what they're doing. Or just being there and being present instead of constantly worrying about where the fetal heart is instead of focusing on how they're labouring and talking them through, you know what I mean? (p. 390)

Coddington and colleagues (2023) have also interviewed fifteen women who used the "beltless" system to understand their experiences of it. It is important to note that all the women in this study were considered to be at increased risk and had been advised to have CTG monitoring, and most were aiming to avoid the use of an epidural and to remain active in labour. Their experiences with the "beltless" system might not be the same for other women with different priorities.

Women in this study reported wearing the sensors was very comfortable: "You don't really notice it's there… it's just one less thing that you really had to think about" (p. 548). The "beltless" system made it easier to move about in labour and women spoke of how this helped them feel more in control and like an active participant in their labour. One of the women said:

> I think in a high risk pregnancy particularly… you feel very micro-managed and it's quite medicalised and so just having something to be able to have control over or a little bit of freedom to be able to make a choice [of position] during the labour process, it was quite nice. (p. 549).

While the beltless system required less "fiddling" to maintain the CTG recording than standard CTG sensors, there were some women who did need to have the sensors repositioned during labour. One woman said:

> I did just find a couple of issues ... the top sticker kept coming off. It wasn't fully removing itself [but] it wasn't picking up what it needed to pick up all the time. There was a lot of my midwife running in, trying to re-stick it and try to leave me in peace and then running back in, trying to re-stick it, leaving me in peace. (p. 550).

"Beltless" systems are now available for hospitals to purchase, so you might be able to access one for your own labour. It is important to bear in mind that while "beltless" systems improve comfort and the consistency of the CTG tracing, there has not yet been any research showing this translates into better health outcomes for women and their babies.

How knowledge about fetal heart rate patterns happened in the past

Before I do more looking to the future – let's first sneak a peek back to the past, to illustrate how we came to know some of what we know about fetal heart rate patterns. Edward Hon, an obstetrician, is responsible for much of the early research that set up our understanding of how to make sense of the wiggly lines seen on a CTG trace. Back in 1958, he was recording fetal heart rate patterns during labour and noted that for some women, the fetal heart rate slowed during contractions and returned to where it started from as the contraction ended. We now call this an *early deceleration*. Hon decided these changes were probably due to pressure on the head of the fetus as it pushed against the woman's cervix, rather than being due to low oxygen levels.

Hon tested his theory by performing an experiment on a number of women in labour. He didn't say how many women. He also didn't say whether these women agreed to this experiment. The research was done at a time when deep sedation during labour was common, so it is possible the women had no idea what he was up to. Doing research without permission is seriously unethical! The fact that this research was done, published, and became the basis of clinical practice says a lot about how women were viewed by obstetricians in the late 1950s.

Hon took different sized rings (pessaries designed to treat vaginal prolapse), put one in the woman's vagina, and pushed the ring up firmly against the head of the fetus. For some (but not all) women, the fetal heart rate slowed and returned to where it started from once he took the pressure off.

This is how the story of early decelerations being due to head compression was created. It's hardly definitive science.

Hon later teamed up with another obstetrician, Lee, and in 1963 they published the results of another experiment designed to develop knowledge about changes in the fetal heart rate. This time the research was done on fetuses of women having caesarean section. These women would probably have had a general anaesthetic and again they didn't explain in the paper whether they asked women for permission to do what they did. Once the woman's uterus was open, but before the fetus was lifted out, they attached sensors to the fetus to record the heart rate and blood pressure, then pulled out a loop of umbilical cord and compressed it to study how the fetus responded. Once they had done this a few times, they delivered the baby. (Again, this research would now be considered unethical.)

This study was largely responsible for what maternity professionals are still taught today about another type of deceleration – the variable deceleration. The teaching is that variable decelerations are due to cord compression, and they happen because receptors called baroreceptors sense a drop in blood pressure. Variable decelerations in the fetal heart rate are the most common type of deceleration seen during labour. In current guidelines about fetal heart rate monitoring, variable decelerations are not considered to be a sign of a serious problem until they happen over a long period of time or there are other changes in the heart rate to suggest that there is a problem.

New understandings of how the fetal heart rate changes

Whizz forward in time, and we encounter a team of physiology researchers who are now updating our understanding of how the fetal heart rate responds to different events that can occur during labour. They have looked at all the research on why early decelerations happen and shown that the idea they are due to head compression is, well, nonsense (Lear, et al., 2023). Instead, early decelerations, like all other types of decelerations, are a response to low oxygen levels designed to protect the fetus from damage by reducing the amount of oxygen needed to keep the heart functioning (Lear, et al., 2018).

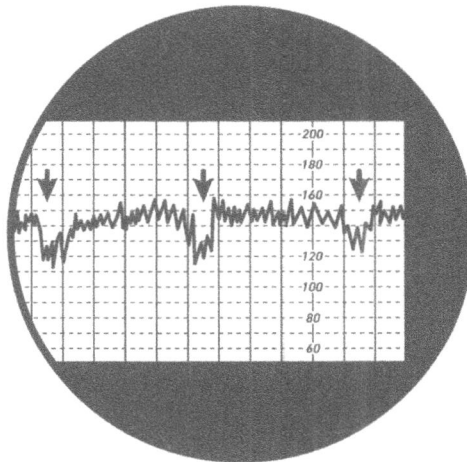

Three decelerations in a CTG recording

They have also looked at the older research about variable decelerations and cord compression. Then they did their own tests on sheep (Lear, et al., 2016). Using pregnant sheep as research subjects means that researchers can deliberately produce low oxygen levels that fall into the harmful range, something that would never be acceptable in human research. They wrote:

> There is strikingly little evidence to support this concept [that cord compression causes variable decelerations by activating baroreceptors]. Umbilical cord compression can occur in labour, for example, during entanglements of the cord or cord prolapse, albeit there is no empirical evidence that it is the predominant cause of fetal heart rate decelerations in the majority of labours. (p. 4174)

In other words, yes, cord compression can occur, but variable decelerations are common and there's nothing to suggest that when variable decelerations happen, they are always caused by cord compression.

This is an important point. If what we thought was true about fetal heart rate patterns isn't true, and professional teaching about this hasn't caught up with what is true, then it isn't hard to see why fetal heart rate monitoring hasn't been able to prevent death or injury.

It remains possible that physiology researchers might yet identify heart rate patterns that really do tell us when the fetus has low oxygen levels and isn't doing okay. In their 2016 paper, Lear and his team suggested we should ignore the shape and timing of the deceleration (and therefore not call them early, variable, or late decelerations) and instead focus on the amount of time the fetal heart rate is lower than what is the average heart rate for this fetus, and how low the heart rate drops. There is a small amount of research showing that this approach performs better than previous approaches to interpreting

CTG recordings for identifying babies born with signs they were exposed to low oxygen levels shortly before birth (Cahill et al., 2018; Cohen et al., 2023; Geva et al., 2023; Talmor et al., 2023). Whether using this new approach will lead to better outcomes for babies, or avoid unnecessary surgical birth, we don't yet know as that research has not yet been done.

New developments in computer interpretation of the CTG

Back in chapter six, I wrote about the use of computers to interpret the CTG recording. It was hoped that training computers to read the CTG would achieve consistency in interpretation and lead to better outcomes. As discussed in that chapter, computer interpretation of the CTG has not (yet) shown improved outcomes compared to having maternity professionals interpret the CTG.

The first systems providing computer interpretation of CTG recordings were trained by human experts. Computer programs were written that could "see" patterns that were the same as when human experts looked at them. While computer interpretation provides consistent interpretation (the same shape of wiggle will be called the same thing every time) this will only lead to better outcomes if knowledge about what produces the fetal heart rate patterns the computer is detecting is correct. As I just explained, there is evidence to suggest that we don't have this bit right.

Given that we humans haven't worked out the precise heart rate patterns that tell us the fetus would benefit from being born right now, researchers have started letting computers train themselves in CTG interpretation. Rather than having human experts tell them what to make of patterns that can be seen with human eyes, machine learning, or artificial intelligence, is used (Knupp et al., 2020). To do this, large databanks containing a lot of CTG recordings are used, where the outcome for the baby is known. The computer examines data from the recordings where the baby was healthy, and those where the baby was not healthy, and looks for changes that humans might not be able to see that can tell the two apart.

This has led to (among other possibilities) a measure known as the fetal stress index. Preliminary research in 493 women showed the fetal stress index can predict babies who will be born with high acid levels in their blood (Gatellier et al, 2020). We do not yet know whether using the fetal stress index will translate into better outcomes for women and their babies.

It is possible that computers might see something we humans can't see, and this could radically transform the way CTG recordings are interpreted. While this sounds great at first glance, I (and others like Begley et al., 2020) have concerns about the unintended consequences of widespread adoption of artificial intelligence systems for fetal heart rate monitoring in labour. With artificial intelligence systems, woman would be largely left out of the conversation occurring between the CTG technology and the maternity professional. Artificial intelligence might reinforce the attitude that women's ideal role in birth is to be a passive, unquestioning, baby producing "machine".

Bjerring and Busch (2021) call systems like computer interpretation of the CTG a "black-box artificial intelligence system" because you can't see what is going on inside the box. There would simply be no way for a human viewer to understand what the computer is seeing. Bjerring and Busch explained their concern that because black-box systems:

> do not reveal ... how or why they reach the recommendations that they do, then neither can practitioners who rely on these black-box systems in decision making ... explain to patients how and why they give the recommendations they do. Yet for patients to make decisions in autonomous and rational ways, it is a requirement that they have the capacity to make sense of the medical information presented and can process it rationally to reach a decision that furthers their health care goals. (p. 361)

The risk then, is that when a woman is advised to have intervention in her labour because of a concern about the fetal heart rate of her unborn baby, no further information is available other than something along the lines of "the computer says so". How can you make a rational decision in this situation? Not only should we be questioning whether we *could* introduce artificial intelligence technology for fetal heart rate monitoring, we need to ask whether we should introduce it in practice.

The unsolvable problem of fetal heart rate monitoring

There are several assumptions that must be true for fetal heart rate monitoring (of any sort) to prevent injury to the fetus during labour. These assumptions are:

✧ A fetus with low oxygen levels will have a recognisable change in its heart rate pattern

✧ A fetus with low oxygen levels and an abnormal heart rate pattern has not already developed irreversible damage but is likely to

✧ There is a window of time when it is possible for maternity professionals to do something that can either return oxygen levels to normal, or achieve the birth of the baby, before irreversible damage happens

✧ All (or almost all) fetuses with one of these recognised abnormal patterns have low oxygen levels.

While there is research showing that babies who are born with health issues due to low oxygen levels were more likely to have abnormal heart rate patterns in labour, these patterns were also common in healthy babies (Reynolds et al., 2022). Let me show you what that looks like, and why it is so hard to use the presence of an abnormal heart rate as a predictor for poor health. In the study by Reynolds and his team, 60% of babies with brain injury had a properly very abnormal heart rate pattern (called pathological in the guideline they used for interpretation). In babies who were healthy at birth, 26% also had a pathological heart rate pattern.

At first glance that makes it look like a midwife or doctor who is looking at a pathological heart rate pattern can tell this is a baby with a problem two times out of three. But that's not how the maths actually works out. Moderate to severe hypoxic ischaemic encephalopathy, the type of brain injury included in this study, affects about one baby in 1,000 (Chakkarapani et al., 2025). Let's say that a busy city hospital provides care for 5,000 women who go into labour each year and everyone uses CTG monitoring. Five of those women will give birth to a baby with this particular brain injury. If 60% of these women have a pathological CTG, that is three women. On the other hand, 4,995 women will give birth to a baby who does not have this brain injury, and 26% of them will have a pathological CTG. That is 1,299 women. In total, 1,302 women will have a pathological CTG. Only a tiny 0.2% of women with a pathological CTG will have a baby that is being damaged by low oxygen levels, and 99.8% will not. Trying to guess which of the 1,302 women have a baby that might benefit from earlier birth, and which will not, is simply impossible.

Understanding the physiology of fetal heart responses to low oxygen

A major problem with all types of fetal heart rate monitoring is that researchers haven't yet proven accurately which heart rate patterns differentiate between "my oxygen levels are low but I'm coping just fine" and one that means "my oxygen is low, and it would be good to get out of here soon". It is important to keep in mind that these heart rate changes are about protection from damage rather than communicating "distress" to a maternity professional. For most mammals over the course of evolution, there was no external source of help to rescue a fetus, so the mammals that survived to pass their genes on were those with well-developed self-protective mechanisms. Brief, repeated falls in oxygen levels, over the duration of labour are part of the picture of most labours, and the overwhelming majority of fetuses are really good at managing this.

Lear's team of physiology researchers have shown that what is doing much of this protection is a thing called the peripheral chemoreceptor reflex. It looks like this. Falling levels of oxygen in body tissues are detected by chemoreceptors and trigger multiple responses. The heart rate slows. The heart requires oxygen to produce each heartbeat, so fewer beats per minute reduces the amount of oxygen it needs. This fall in workload, seen as a deceleration, protects heart cells from damage. Decelerations are an easily recognisable change seen when fetal heart rate monitoring is used in labour – whether that is intermittent auscultation or CTG monitoring.

Other things are happening too. Blood vessels around the body of the fetus squeeze tight. This reduces the amount of blood going to toes, ears, the gut, and so on – parts of the body that are not essential for immediate survival. Blood shifts to the brain and the heart instead. These are the two most essential organs and they both need a lot of oxygen to function properly. We can't see or measure this shift with fetal heart rate monitoring, but that doesn't mean it isn't happening.

There's a big problem with using decelerations to distinguish between the "leave me alone, I'm fine" fetus and the "get me out now" fetus. The peripheral chemoreceptor reflex behaves the same way in both of these lower oxygen situations (Lear et al., 2018). The reflex doesn't change over time as oxygen levels fall even lower and damage starts to occur. So a fetus who is coping fine will have a fetal heart rate pattern that looks the same as a fetus who is no longer coping.

Changes in fetal behaviour also occur when oxygen levels fall. Active movement requires oxygen, so the fetus with low oxygen levels is going to move less to conserve this oxygen. Four behavioural states can be identified on ultrasound, namely quiet sleep, active sleep, quiet awake, and active awake (Stone, et al., 2017). While these states can't be seen directly on a CTG recording, there are clues in the average heart rate (or baseline) and the degree of change in the heart rate over a short period of time (known as heart rate variability) that can help to guess the behavioural state for that fetus at that time. With lower oxygen, quiet sleep and quiet awake patterns are more common.

Maternity professionals use information about the baseline and fetal heart rate variability as part of their assessment of fetal heart rate patterns, in addition to using decelerations, to help tell the difference between the "leave me alone" and "get me out now" fetus. While that sounds like it might solve our problem, there's been very little research to understand whether changes in heart rate variability can differentiate between these two states (Tournier et al., 2021). There really are huge gaps in our knowledge about how to understand what is happening when different fetal heart rate patterns occur in labour. This knowledge gap means the assumptions I listed at the start of this section remain as unproven beliefs rather than facts.

So – here's my belief. Perhaps I will eventually be proven wrong, but my belief is based on having studied this area for many years. It is this:

> We will never reduce birth complications from low oxygen supply in labour by continuing to use fetal heart rate monitoring as our main tool.

I mean all forms of fetal heart rate monitoring. From the low-tech Pinard used to listen to the fetal heart rate, to the fanciest, wireless, "beltless", artificial intelligence backed, technology solution that looks all shiny and bright. That's possibly a pretty depressing thought to find at the end of an entire book about fetal heart rate monitoring. I believe the key to finding a better approach lies in being honest that what we have been doing for the past 60 years doesn't – and won't ever – work. Being honest about the situation should mean that research and development funding gets shifted to finding new solutions, rather than focussing on making CTG monitoring more comfortable for women, or easier for maternity professionals to work with.

I have been keeping an eye on the development of types of fetal monitoring that use something other than the heart rate, as these might be the key to finally finding an approach that really delivers on the promise that it will prevent unnecessary heart ache for families from the loss of a healthy child.

Transabdominal fetal oximetry

All the technologies described so far have aimed to show whether fetal oxygen levels are okay or not by using an approach other than measuring oxygen directly. It is possible to measure fetal oxygen saturation levels directly (Garite et al., 2000). This is called fetal oximetry.

Oxygen saturation is the percentage of haemoglobin molecules in red blood cells that have an oxygen molecule attached. To measure this, a long narrow sensor probe is inserted through the woman's vagina, so the monitoring device lies alongside the cheek of her fetus. Light is generated by the probe and it bounces off the tissues underneath it with some being absorbed, and some reflected back to the sensor. The colour of the reflected light is used to indicate oxygen saturation. It is similar to the technology used in the finger probes used to measure oxygen saturation in adults.

A Cochrane review (East et al., 2014) has compared the use of fetal oximetry in labour in addition to CTG monitoring rather than CTG monitoring alone. No differences in outcomes for the baby or in the caesarean or instrumental birth rates were noted. No research has ever compared fetal oximetry on its own (without also using a CTG at the same time) with either CTG monitoring or intermittent auscultation.

Unlike the other technologies described thus far, fetal oximetry probes are no longer commercially available. These sensors never really took off in practice, in part because they needed to be placed inside the woman's uterus. The real game changer is being able to monitor fetal and placental oxygen levels using sensors placed externally on the woman's abdomen (Fong et al., 2020; Kang et al., 2021; Kasap et al., 2024).

We have a long way to go before trans-abdominal fetal oximetry turns up on a birth suite near you. Before it does, we need rigorous research to show whether or not using it (either alone or in combination with some form of fetal heart rate monitoring) improves outcomes for the fetus. It is also important that researchers ask women about their experiences with the new technology so we aren't imposing something harmful on them, and that we examine the long-term outcome of hours of exposure to near infra-red light (the technology used to measure the oxygen levels) in utero.

Who knows whether this might end up being a better approach than either CTG monitoring or intermittent auscultation. It does make sense to me that if you want to know about oxygen levels, then actually measuring oxygen levels is a better approach than trying to guess what they are by measuring something else.

Fetal brain waves

Assessing brain function might be another approach worth investing in. The brain generates many tiny electrical impulses as part of its normal functioning. When oxygen levels falls, brain activity becomes quieter to conserve the precious oxygen. These electrical signals can be recorded by sensors placed on the scalp. This is known as electroencephalography or EEG, and there are well developed systems in use for children and adults.

A team of researchers from the UK and Slovenia have been experimenting with an interesting way to record the EEG from a fetus during labour (Mires, et al., 2022). They have made use of existing technology: the fetal spiral electrode and an EEG recording system. To see if the idea might be worth looking into, they applied fetal spiral electrodes to the scalps of 18 healthy adult volunteers. And yes, they could record the EEG this way.

In theory then, with perhaps some modifications, it might be possible to continuously record the fetal EEG during labour to monitor how brain function changes over time. The downsides of fetal spiral electrode use would remain an issue (like the discomfort of insertion for the woman, reducing her mobility, and risk of infection or trauma to the fetal skin). And there is a long way to go in terms of understanding what the EEG patterns in labour mean. But it might move us closer towards a monitoring technology that helps maternity professionals step in and interrupt the processes of labour when, and only when, doing so will mean better outcomes for the baby.

What would an ideal fetal monitoring technology look like?

Measuring oxygen levels or EEG patterns could be a way to monitor the health of the baby in labour without using heart rate patterns. One of these, or perhaps some entirely new way of monitoring, might mean we can finally prevent uncommon harms to the fetus during labour from low oxygen levels. Here's my wish list for what a future technology would look like.

✧ It would be accurate. All fetuses with dangerously low levels of oxygen would be identified, and all fetuses with adequate oxygen levels would register a normal reading.

✧ It would work for babies. We would have solid research showing that using the new monitor prevented death and organ damage from low oxygen during labour. The research would include long term follow up as well as short term studies.

✧ It would work for women. The technology would be minimally intrusive and allow women to do whatever they need or want to do during labour. It would not require vaginal examinations and opening of the membranes.

✧ It would not lead to unintended harm for either the baby or the woman. As well as research showing that the monitor worked, researchers would also have carefully checked to make sure it wasn't creating new problems.

✧ It would work for maternity professionals. The technology would be easy to use, and not require lots of fiddling, or hours of study and regular educational updates to be able to use it properly. It would not add unnecessarily to professionals' workload or prevent them from remaining focused on the overall wellbeing of the woman and her fetus.

✧ It would be designed with, rather than for, the people who will use it. Women and their family members; and midwives, nurses, and obstetricians would be involved early on in the development of the technology. The technology would be designed to enhance women's active participation in decision making rather than reinforce beliefs that women don't get to decide. It would overcome, rather than reinforce, harmful cultural forces in maternity services that maintain traditional battle lines between doctors, nurses, and midwives.

◇ It would be cost effective, sustainable, and available to everyone who wanted to use it, even in low-income countries.

◇ It would be environmentally sound, not generating large amounts of waste or using a lot of electricity to operate.

Final thoughts

If you are pregnant and making decisions about fetal heart rate monitoring for your upcoming labour, there is no magic solution the promises a great outcome. While that is frustrating, it does reflect the reality of many other things in our lives. Decision making is always about doing the best you can, with what you have, at the time you are making your decision.

I am confident you will make the right decisions for you.

I said at the start of this book that my position is that CTGs are nonsense. Believing the inaccurate hype about CTG use might reduce anxiety and lead to a (false but comforting) sense of safety. Knowing about the reality of fetal heart rate monitoring can take away that sense of security. Throughout obstetric history, women have been told not to worry their pretty heads about bad stuff. That's never been alright, and it isn't alright now.

Women want more from their maternity services. Knowing the reality of the situation may be uncomfortable, but ultimately makes for better decision making. Knowing the reality opens the possibility of changing maternity services so they meet women's needs. Knowing the reality opens up opportunities for researchers to finally develop an approach that actually works.

Glossary

Apgar score A score given out of ten based on the baby's heart rate, skin colour, breathing, muscle tone, and reflex movements. Typically measured at one and five minutes of age. A low score (usually defined as less than seven) generally suggests that additional support with breathing would be of benefit.

Cardiotocograph (CTG) A device used to record the fetal heart rate (cardio), the activity of the woman's uterus (toco), that plots both these pieces of information on a graph over time. Also commonly referred to as an electronic fetal monitor.

Central fetal monitoring Digital information from CTG recordings is displayed on monitors in locations outside the room where the woman is given birth. Information from all women using CTG monitoring in the birth suite is visible from the central fetal monitoring area.

Cerebral palsy A permanent form of brain injury that can lead to a collection of problems like abnormal movements, blindness, deafness, speech disorders, and learning disabilities. There are many causes of cerebral palsy, with brain injury during labour considered to be a small contributor.

Cochrane Library A collection of systematic literature reviews of randomised controlled trials about healthcare issues. All the reviews use the same specific approach to finding, analysing, and describing research. This approach is considered to generate high quality information about healthcare interventions to guide clinical practice. The Library is available online – https://www.cochranelibrary.com

Doppler A form of ultrasound used to monitor blood flow. Sound waves are bounced off moving structures inside the body and the reflected sound is measured to detect a change in frequency called the Doppler effect. Doppler technology is used in handheld portable fetal monitoring devices and the external sensors used for CTG monitoring.

Electrocardiograph (ECG) A device used to record electric activity generated by the heart. This information can be used to count the heart rate or to look for changes in the pattern of electrical activity that suggest injury to the heart.

Fetal blood sampling The process of collecting a small sample of blood from the fetus during labour. The blood can be tested to measure general levels of acid (pH) or one specific type of acid (lactate). Fetal blood sampling aims to provide more information to maternity professionals when the fetal heart rate pattern is abnormal.

Fetal heart rate monitoring Any approach used to gather information about the fetal heart rate and interpret the heart rate to understand whether it is considered normal or not, with the aim of improving health outcomes for that fetus / baby.

Fetal oximetry A way of testing the amount of oxygen in the fetal blood blood. A sensor placed on the skin of the fetus pulses light into the skin. The colour of the light reflected back is measured and the difference between the light going in and the light coming back is used to indicate how much oxygen is in the blood.

Fetal spiral electrode A fetal spiral electrode is used to detect the fetal ECG pattern. They are used for internal CTG monitoring. The electrode must pass through the woman's vagina to be attached to the fetus. Often referred to as a scalp clip.

Fetus The name given to a baby during pregnancy.

Hypoxic ischaemic encephalopathy (HIE) Signs of brain injury that happens before, during, or soon after birth, caused by low oxygen levels in the brain (hypoxia) and / or reduced blood flow to the brain (ischaemia). Signs include high levels of acid in the blood, seizures, breathing problems, low muscle tone, and others. Hypoxic ischaemic encephalopathy is graded mild, moderate, or severe. Some babies make a full recovery, while others go on to have permanent brain injury.

Intermittent auscultation A form of fetal heart rate monitoring that involves listening (auscultating) the fetal heart rate for a short period of time, repeated regularly during labour. A handheld Doppler device is often used, or a Pinard or something similar.

Intrauterine pressure catheter A long thin tube inserted through the woman's vagina into the woman's uterus and used to measure the pressure inside the uterus. This provides a way to monitoring the timing, duration, and strength of her contractions.

Lactate A byproduct of breaking down glucose (sugar) molecules to generate energy, particularly when oxygen levels are low. Lactate levels can be measured in blood and provide a rough indication that oxygen levels have recently been low.

Maternity professional A person who works to provide care to women and their babies during pregnancy, birth, and the first few weeks after birth. They have completed specific officially recognised training programs required for their role. They are likely to be registered by a government agency that oversees professional standards and may require proof that they stay up to date with the knowledge required to practice safely. Maternity professionals include midwives, nurses, obstetricians, and others.

Meconium stained liquor Meconium is the name given to the first bowel movement produce by the baby. When this is passed before birth, it is mixed into the liquor (or amniotic fluid – the fluid around the fetus inside the uterus) and produces a distinct greenish colour. One of the reasons why this happens is low oxygen levels prior to birth.

Meta-analysis A way to summarise the findings from multiple sources of research. It is used when comparing studies that used the same intervention (for example CTG use) and the same control (for example intermittent auscultation) that measured the same outcome (for example death).

Neonatal mortality A measure of the number of deaths occurring in the first 28 days of life. Early neonatal mortality measures deaths in the first week of life.

Non-invasive fetal ECG (NifECG) A form of CTG monitoring that uses sensors attached externally on the woman's abdomen to detect the fetal ECG and electrical activity from the woman's uterus. Also called "beltless" CTG monitoring as the sensors use adhesive to attach to the skin rather than the straps used with other external forms of CTG monitoring.

Oxytocin A hormone that causes uterine contractions to occur and become stronger and longer. Given as an intravenous infusion to induce labour, or during labour to make contractions stronger and more frequent.

Perinatal mortality A measure of the number of deaths of the fetus / baby occurring during during pregnancy (stillbirth) and up to 28 days after birth.

Pinard A type of stethoscope designed for listening to the fetal heart.

Randomised controlled trial A type of research used to compare an intervention against a control (either no intervention or another intervention). Research participants are randomly divided up to have either the intervention or the control. This approach reduces the possibility that the results of the research are due to something other than the intervention being tested.

Risk assessment An approach used in healthcare (and other) systems to identify groups of people who are more likely to develop a poor healthcare outcome. People are then divided into low and high risk groups. Once risks are identified, risk management approaches can be used.

Risk management A series of approaches used in healthcare (and other) systems in an attempt to reduce the chance of poor health outcomes. This can include the use of additional tests, medications, surgical procedures, or other forms of care aimed at reducing the chance of a poor outcome.

Seizures Abnormal jerky movements of the arms, legs, and body. They are typically due to irritation or damage to parts of the brain that control movement. Seizures soon after birth can be a sign of brain injury due to low oxygen levels but can also be caused by other things, like withdrawal from certain drugs.

Stethoscope A device used to amplify sounds from inside the body and transfer the sound to the ear of a person listening to those sounds.

Stillbirth The death of the fetus prior to birth. Definitions vary from one country to the next. A common definition is the death of the fetus at or after 20 weeks of pregnancy. (Earlier deaths are classified as miscarriages.)

ST segment analysis (STAN) Analysis of the shape of the fetal ECG pattern, generally done using computer software. STAN aims to identify changes in the fetal ECG that are believed to show low levels of oxygen affecting the fetal heart rate. It can be used as an additional test alongside CTG monitoring.

Systematic review A structured approach to collecting, analysing, and describing findings from more than one piece of research. Systematic reviews are designed to gather all the relevant information on a particular topic in order to answer one or more research questions.

Telemetry A form of CTG monitoring that uses transmitters to communicate information from sensors recording either or both the fetal heart rate and the woman's uterine activity to the CTG monitor, without the use of wires. Also called "wireless" CTG monitoring.

References

Alfirevic, Z., Devane, D., Gyte, G., & Cuthbert, A. (2017). Continuous cardiotocography (CTG) as a form of electronic fetal monitoring (EFM) for fetal assessment during labour. *Cochrane Database of Systematic Reviews, 2(CD006066), 1-137.* http://doi.wiley.com/10.1002/14651858.CD006066.pub3

Al Wattar, B., Lakhiani, A., Sacco, A., Siddharth, A., Bain, A., Calvia, A., Kamran, A., ... & AB-FAB study group. (2019). Evaluating the value of intrapartum fetal scalp blood sampling to predict adverse neonatal outcomes: A UK multicentre observational study. *European Journal of Obstetrics, Gynecology & Reproductive Biology, 240, 62-67.* https://linkinghub.elsevier.com/retrieve/pii/S0301211519302982

Andriani, R., Safari, M., Hidayat, Y., Husin, F., Nugraha, G., Susiarno, H., & Cahyadi, W. (2018). Mixed juice consumption during labour to the mother's blood lactate levels. *Global Medical & Health Communication, 6(3), 169-175.* https://doi.org/10.29313/gmhc.v6i3.2907

Annandale, E., Baston, H., Beynon-Jones, S., Brierley-Jones, L., Brodrick, A., Chappell, P., Green, J., Jackson, C., Land, V., & Stacey, T. (2022). *In Shared decision-making during childbirth in maternity units: the VIP mixed-methods study.* https://www.ncbi.nlm.nih.gov/pubmed/36534749

American College of Obstetricians and Gynecologists. (2009). *Intrapartum fetal heart rate monitoring: Nomenclature, interpretation, and general management principles. ACOG Practice Bulletin Number 106.* https://journals.lww.com/greenjournal/citation/2009/07000/acog_practice_bulletin_no__106__intrapartum_fetal.51.aspx

American College of Obstetricians and Gynecologists. (2019). ACOG Committee Opinion Number 766: Approaches to limit intervention during labor and birth. *Obstetrics & Gynecology, 133, e164-e173.* https://doi.org/10.1097/AOG.0000000000003074

Ampt, A., Patterson, J., Roberts, C., & Ford, J. (2015). Obstetric anal sphincter injury rates among primiparous women with different modes of vaginal delivery. *International Journal of Gynecology & Obstetrics, 131(3), 260-264.* http://doi.wiley.com/10.1016/j.ijgo.2015.06.025

Amyx, M., Philibert, M., Farr, A., Donati, S., Smarason, A. K., Tica, V., Velebil, P., Alexander, S., Durox, M., Elorriaga, M. F., Heller, G., Kyprianou, T., Mierzejewska, E., Verdenik, I., Zile-Velika, I., Zeitlin, J., & the Euro-Peristat Research Group. (2024). Trends in caesarean section rates in Europe from 2015 to 2019 using Robson's Ten Group Classification System: A Euro-Peristat study. *BJOG, 131(4), 444-454.* https://doi.org/10.1111/1471-0528.17670

Argyridis, S., & Arulkumaran, S. (2016). Meconium stained amniotic fluid. *Obstetrics, Gynaecology & Reproductive Medicine, 26(8), 227-230.* http://dx.doi.org/10.1016/j.ogrm.2016.05.001

Asta, A., Ghi, T., Pedrazzi, G., & Frusca, T. (2016). Does vacuum delivery carry a higher risk of shoulder dystocia? Review and meta-analysis of the literature. *European Journal of Obstetrics, Gynecology & Reproductive Biology, 204, 62-68.* http://dx.doi.org/10.1016/j.ejogrb.2016.07.506

Australian Institute of Health and Welfare. (2025). *Australia's mothers and babies.* https://www.aihw.gov.au/reports-data/population-groups/mothers-babies/overview

Ayres-de-Campos, D., Spong, C. Y., Chandraharan, E., & Panel for the FIGO Intrapartum Fetal Monitoring Expert Consensus Panel. (2015). FIGO consensus guidelines on intrapartum fetal monitoring: Cardiotocography. *International Journal of Gynecology & Obstetrics, 131(1), 13-24.* https://doi.org/10.1016/j.ijgo.2015.06.020

Bakkar, J., Verhoeven, C., Janssen, P., van Lith, J., van Oudgaarden, E., Bloemenkamp, K., Papatsonis, D., Mol, B., & van der Post, J. (2010). Outcomes after internal versus external tocodynamometry for monitoring labor. *New England Journal of Medicine, 362, 306-313.* https://www.nejm.org/doi/full/10.1056/NEJMoa0902748

Baumfeld, Y., Sheiner, E., Wainstock, T., Segal, I., Sergienko, R., Landau, D., & Walfisch, A. (2018). Elective cesarean delivery at term and the long-term risk for neurological morbidity of the offspring. *American Journal of Perinatology, 35(11), 1038-1043*. https://www.ncbi.nlm.nih.gov/pubmed/29510422

Begley, K., Begley, C., & Smith, V. (2020). Shared decision-making and maternity care in the deep learning age: Acknowledging and overcoming inherited defeaters. *Journal of Evaluation in Clinical Practice, 27(3), 497-503*. https://www.ncbi.nlm.nih.gov/pubmed/33188540

Ben M'Barek, I., Jauvion, G., & Ceccaldi, P. F. (2022). Computerized cardiotocography analysis during labor - A state-of-the-art review. *Acta Obstetrica et Gynecologica Scandinavica, 102(2), 130-137*. https://doi.org/10.1111/aogs.14498

Bjerring, J., & Busch, J. (2021). Artificial intelligence and patient-centred decision making. *Philosophy & Technology, 34, 349-371*. https://doi.org/10.1007/s13347-019-00391-6

Blix, E., Brurberg, K., Reierth, E., Reinar, L., & Oian, P. (2024). ST waveform analysis vs cardiotocography alone for intrapartum fetal monitoring: An updated systematic review and meta-analysis of randomized trials. *Acta Obstetrica et Gynecologica Scandanavica, 103(3), 437-448*. https://doi.org/10.1111/aogs.14752

Blix, E., Eskild, A., Skau, I., & Grytten, J. (2022). The impact of the introduction of intrapartum fetal ECG ST segment analysis. A population study. *Acta Obstetricia et Gynecologica Scandinavica, 101(7), 809-818*. https://doi.org/10.1111/aogs.14347

Blix, E., & Öhlund, L. (2007). Norwegian midwives' perception of the labour admission test. *Midwifery, 23(1), 48-58*. https://doi.org/10.1016/j.midw.2005.10.003

Bodner, K., Wierrani, F., Grünberger, W., & Bodner-Adler, B. (2010). Influence of the mode of delivery on maternal and neonatal outcomes: a comparison between elective cesarean section and planned vaginal delivery in a low-risk obstetric population. *Archives of Gynecology & Obstetrics, 283(6), 1193-1198*. http://link.springer.com/10.1007/s00404-010-1525-y

Bovbjerg, M., Dissanayake, M. V., Cheyney, M., Brown, J., & Snowden, J. (2019). Utility of the 5-minute Apgar score as a research endpoint. *American Journal of Epidemiology, 188(9), 1695-1704*. https://doi.org/10.1093/aje/kwz132

Brimacombe, M., Iffy, L., Apuzzio, J., Varadi, V., Nagy, B., Raju, V., & Portuondo, N. (2008). Shoulder dystocia related fetal neurological injuries: the predisposing roles of forceps and ventouse extractions. *Archives of Gynecology & Obstetrics, 277(5), 415-422.* https://www.ncbi.nlm.nih.gov/pubmed/17906870

Brown, J., McIntyre, A., Gasparotto, R., & McGee, T. (2016). Birth outcomes, intervention frequency, and the disappearing midwife-potential hazards of central fetal monitoring: a single center review. *Birth, 43(2), 100-107.* http://doi.wiley.com/10.1111/birt.12222

Cahill, A., Tuuli, M., Stout, M., López, J., & Macones, G. (2018). A prospective cohort study of fetal heart rate monitoring: deceleration area is predictive of fetal acidemia. *American Journal of Obstetrics & Gynecology, 218(5), 523.e521-523.e512.* https://www.ncbi.nlm.nih.gov/pubmed/29408586

Campbell, S. (2013). A short history of sonography in obstetrics and gynaecology. *Facts, Views and Vision in ObGyn, 5(3), 213-229.* https://www.ncbi.nlm.nih.gov/pubmed/24753947

Chakkarapani, E., de Vries, L., Ferriero, D. M., & Gunn, A. (2025). Neonatal encephalopathy and hypoxic-ischemic encephalopathy: the state of the art. *Pediatric Research, in press.* https://doi.org/10.1038/s41390-025-03986-2

Chan, W., Paul, R., & Toews, J. (1973). Intrapartum fetal monitoring. Maternal and fetal morbidity and perinatal mortality. *Obstetrics & Gynecology, 41(1), 7-13.* https://www.ncbi.nlm.nih.gov/pubmed/4682619

Chua, S., Kurup, A., Arulkumaran, S., & Ratnam, S. (1990). Augmentation of labor: Does internal tocography result in better obstetric outcome than external tocography? *Obstetrics & Gynecology, 76, 164-167.* https://www.ncbi.nlm.nih.gov/pubmed/2196493

Chuey, M., De Vries, R., Dal Cin, S., & Low, L. (2020). Maternity providers' perspectives on barriers to utilization of intermittent fetal monitoring: A qualitative study. *Journal of Perinatal & Neonatal Nursing, 34(1), 46-55.* https://doi.org/10.1097/JPN.0000000000000453

Coddington, R., Scarf, V., & Fox, D. (2023). Australian women's experiences of wearing a non-invasive fetal electrocardiography (NIFECG) device during labour. *Women & Birth, 36(6), 546-551.* https://doi.org/10.1016/j.wombi.2023.03.005

Cohen, G., Ravid, D., Gnaiem, N., Gluska, H., Schreiber, H., Haleluya, N., Biron-Shental, T., Kovo, M., & Markovitch, O. (2023). The impact of total deceleration area and fetal growth on neonatal acidemia in vacuum extraction deliveries. *Children, 10(5)*. https://doi.org/10.3390/children10050776

Cohen, W., & Hayes-Gill, B. (2014). Influence of maternal body mass index on accuracy and reliability of external fetal monitoring techniques. *Acta Obstetricia et Gynecologica Scandinavica, 93(6), 590-595*. http://doi.wiley.com/10.1111/aogs.12387

Cohen, W., Ommani, S., Hassan, S., Mirza, F., Solomon, M., Brown, R., Schifrin, B., Himsworth, J., & Hayes-Gill, B. (2012). Accuracy and reliability of fetal heart rate monitoring using maternal abdominal surface electrodes. *Acta Obstetricia et Gynecologica Scandinavica, 91(11), 1306-1313*. https://doi.org/10.1111/j.1600-0412.2012.01533.x

Cox, L. W. (1961). Foetal distress. *Australian & New Zealand Journal of Obstetrics & Gynaecology, 1(3), 99-103*.

Christie, D., & Tansey, E. (2001). Origins of Neonatal Intensive Care. Wellcome Witnesses to Twentieth Century Medicine. https://histmodbiomed.history.qmul.ac.uk/sites/default/files/44831.pdf

Dahlquist, K., Stuart, A., & Kallen, K. (2022). Planned cesarean section vs planned vaginal delivery among women without formal medical indication for planned cesarean section: A retrospective cohort study of maternal short-term complications. *Acta Obstetrica et Gynecologica Scandinavica, 101(9), 1026-1032*. https://www.ncbi.nlm.nih.gov/pubmed/35841162

Davey, C., & Moore, A. (2006). Necrotizing fasciitis of the scalp in a newborn. *Obstetrics & Gynecology, 107(2), 461-463*. https://www.ncbi.nlm.nih.gov/pubmed/16449149

Declercq, E., Barger, M., Cabral, H., Evans, S., Kotelchuck, M., Simon, C., Weiss, J., & Heffner, L. (2007). Maternal outcomes associated with planned primary cesarean births compared with planned vaginal births. *Obstetrics & Gynecology, 109(3), 669-677*. https://www.ncbi.nlm.nih.gov/pubmed/17329519

de Costa, C. M. (2020). The Pill: A short history. *O&G Magazine, 22(1), 1-22*. https://www.ogmagazine.org.au/22/1-22/the-pill-a-short-history/

Dekker, G., Chan, A., Luke, C., Priest, K., Riley, M., Halliday, J., King, J., Gee, V., O'Neill, M., Snell, M., Cull, V., & Cornes, S. (2010). Risk of uterine rupture in Australian women attempting vaginal birth after one prior caesarean section: a retrospective population-based cohort study. *British Journal of Obstetrics & Gynaecology, 117(11), 1358-1365.* http://doi.wiley.com/10.1111/j.1471-0528.2010.02688.x

Devane, D., Lalor, J., Daly, S., McGuire, W., Cuthbert, A., Smith, V. (2017). Cardiotocography versus intermittent auscultation of fetal heart on admission to labour ward for assessment of fetal wellbeing. *Cochrane Database of Systematic Reviews, 1(3), CD005122.* https://dx.doi.org/10.1002/14651858.cd005122.pub5

Doumouchtsis, S., & Arulkumaran, S. (2008). Head trauma after instrumental births. *Clinics in Perinatology, 35(1), 69-83, viii.* https://www.ncbi.nlm.nih.gov/pubmed/18280876

Dover, S., & Gauge, S. (1995). Fetal monitoring - midwifery attitudes. *Midwifery, 11(1), 18–27.* https://www.ncbi.nlm.nih.gov/pubmed/7731372

Drife, J. O. (2021). The history of labour induction: How did we get here? *Best Practice & Research Clinical Obstetrics & Gynaecology, 77, 3-14.* https://doi.org/10.1016/j.bpobgyn.2021.07.004

D'souza, S., Black, P., Macfarlane, T., & Richardson, B. (1982). Fetal scalp damage and neonatal jaundice: a risk of routine fetal scalp electrode monitoring. *Journal of Obstetrics & Gynaecology, 2(3), 161-164.* http://www.tandfonline.com/doi/full/10.3109/01443618209067698

East, C., Begg, L., Colditz, P., & Lau, R. (2014). Fetal pulse oximetry for fetal assessment in labour. *Cochrane Database of Systematic Reviews, 10, CD004075.* https://www.ncbi.nlm.nih.gov/pubmed/25287809

East, C., Davey, M., Kamlin, C., Davis, P., Sheehan, P., Kane, S., Brennecke, S., & the Flamingo Study Group. (2021). The addition of fetal scalp blood lactate measurement as an adjunct to cardiotocography to reduce caesarean sections during labour: The Flamingo randomised controlled trial. *Australian & New Zealand Journal of Obstetrics & Gynaecology, 61(5), 684-692.* https://www.ncbi.nlm.nih.gov/pubmed/33754338

East, C., Leader, L., Sheehan, P., Henshall, N., Colditz, P., & Lau, R. (2015). Intrapartum fetal scalp lactate sampling for fetal assessment in the presence of a non-reassuring fetal heart rate trace. *Cochrane Database of Systematic Reviews, 5(5), CD006174-CD006174.* https://doi.org/10.1002/14651858. CD006174.pub3

Ellenberg, J., & Nelson, K. (2013). The association of cerebral palsy with birth asphyxia: a definitional quagmire. *Developmental Medicine & Child Neurology, 55(3), 210-216.* https://www.ncbi.nlm.nih.gov/pubmed/23121164

Esteves-Pereira, A., Deneux-Tharaux, C., Nakamura-Pereira, M., Saucedo, M., Bouvier-Colle, M.-H., & Leal, M. (2016). Caesarean delivery and postpartum maternal mortality: A population-based case control study in Brazil. *PLoS ONE, 11(4), e0153396.* http://dx.plos.org/10.1371/journal.pone.0153396

Euliano, T., Darmanjian, S., Nguyen, M., Busowski, J., Euliano, N., & Gregg, A. (2017). Monitoring fetal heart rate during labor: A comparison of three methods. *Journal of Pregnancy, 2017(6), 8529816-8529815.* https://www.ncbi.nlm.nih.gov/pubmed/28392944

Fahmy, W., Crispim, C., & Cliffe, S. (2018) Association between maternal death and cesarean section in Latin America: A systematic literature review. *Midwifery, 59, 88-93.* https://www.ncbi.nlm.nih.gov/pubmed/29421643

Felker, A., Patel, R., Kotnis, R., Kenyon, S., Knight, M., on behalf of MBRRACE-UK. (2024). Saving lives, improving mother's care compiled report – Lessons learned to inform maternity care from the UK and Ireland Confidential Enquiries into Maternal Deaths and Morbidity 2020-2022. National Perinatal Epidemiology Unit. https://www.npeu.ox.ac.uk/mbrrace-uk/reports/maternal-reports/maternal-report-2020-2022

Fergus, P., Hussain, A., Al-Jumeily, D., Huang, D.-S., & Bouguila, N. (2017). Classification of caesarean section and normal vaginal deliveries using foetal heart rate signals and advanced machine learning algorithms. *BioMedical Engineering OnLine, 16, 1-26.* https://www.ncbi.nlm.nih.gov/pubmed/28679415

Fick, T., & Woerdeman, P. A. (2021). Neonatal brain abscess development following fetal scalp electrode placement: a rare complication. *Child's Nervous System, 38(1), 199-202.* https://www.ncbi.nlm.nih.gov/pubmed/33825051

Fitzpatrick, K., Kurinczuk, J., Bhattacharya, S., & Quigley, M. (2019). Planned mode of delivery after previous caesarean section and short-term maternal and perinatal outcomes: A population-based record linkage cohort study in Scotland. *PLOS Medicine, 16(9), e1002913.* https://www.ncbi.nlm.nih.gov/pubmed/31550245

Fong, D., Yamashiro, K., Johnson, M., Vali, K., Galganski, L., Pivetti, C., Farmer, D., Hedriana, H., & Ghiasi, S. (2020). Validation of a novel transabdominal fetal oximeter in a hypoxic fetal lamb model. *Reproductive Sciences, 27(10), 1960-1966.* https://doi.org/10.1007/s43032-020-00215-5

Ford, P., Crowther, S., & Waller, N. (2023). Midwives' experience of personal/professional risk when providing continuity of care to women who decline recommendations: A meta-synthesis of qualitative studies. *Women & Birth, 36(2), e283-e294.* https://doi.org/10.1016/j.wombi.2022.06.014

Fox, A., Glasofer, A., & Long, D. (2022). Time and effort by labor nurses to achieve and maintain a continuous recording of the fetal heart rate via external monitoring. *Nursing for Women's Health, 26(1), 44-50.* https://www.ncbi.nlm.nih.gov/pubmed/35032463

Fox, D., Coddington, R., & Scarf, V. (2022). Wanting to be 'with woman', not with machine: Midwives' experiences of caring for women being continuously monitored in labour. *Women & Birth, 35(4), 387-393.* https://www.ncbi.nlm.nih.gov/pubmed/34556463

Fox, D., Maude, R., Coddington, R., Woodworth, R., Scarf, V., Watson, K., & Foureur, M. (2021). The use of continuous foetal monitoring technologies that enable mobility in labour for women with complex pregnancies: A survey of Australian and New Zealand hospitals. *Midwifery, 93, 102887.* https://www.ncbi.nlm.nih.gov/pubmed/33260005

Frolova, A., Stout, M., Carter, E., Macones, G., Cahill, A., & Raghuraman, N. (2021). Internal fetal and uterine monitoring in obese patients and maternal obstetrical outcomes. *American Journal of Obstetrics & Gynecology MFM, 3(1), 100282.* https://www.ncbi.nlm.nih.gov/pubmed/33451595

Gallimore, I., Matthews, R., Page, G., Smith, L., Fenton, A., Knight, M., Smith, P., Redpath, S., Manktelow, B., on behalf of the MBRRACE-UK Collaboration. (2024). *MBRRACE-UK Perinatal Mortality Surveillance, UK Perinatal Deaths of Babies Born in 2022: State of the Nation Report. Leicester: The Infant Mortality and Morbidity Studies, Department of Population Health Sciences, University of Leicester.* https://timms.le.ac.uk/mbrrace-uk-perinatal-mortality/surveillance/#perinatal-mortality-in-the-uk

Garcia, J., MacDonald, D., Elbourne, D., & Grant, A. (1985). Mothers' views of continuous electronic fetal heart monitoring and intermittent auscultation in a randomized controlled trial. *Birth, 12(2), 79-86.* https://doi.org/10.1111/j.1523-536x.1985.tb00943.x

Garite, T., Dildy, G., McNamara, H., Nageotte, M., Boehm, F., Dellinger, E., Knuppel, R., ... & Swedlow, D. (2000). A multicenter controlled trial of fetal pulse oximetry in the intrapartum management of nonreassuring fetal heart rate patterns. *American Journal of Obstetrics & Gynecology, 183(5), 1049-1058.* https://www.ncbi.nlm.nih.gov/pubmed/11084540

Gatellier, M., De Jonckheere, J., Storme, L., Houfflin-Debarge, V., Ghesquiere, L., & Garabedian, C. (2020). Fetal heart rate variability analysis for neonatal acidosis prediction. *Journal of Clinical Monitoring & Computing, 35(4), 771-777.* https://www.ncbi.nlm.nih.gov/pubmed/32451749

Geva, Y., Yaniv Salem, S., Geva, N., Rotem, R., Talmor, M., Shema, N., Shany, E., & Weintraub, A. Y. (2023). Intrapartum deceleration and acceleration areas are associated with neonatal encephalopathy. *International Journal of Gynaecology & Obstetrics, 161(3), 1061-1068.* https://doi.org/10.1002/ijgo.14638

Goodlin, R. C. (1979). History of fetal monitoring. *American Journal of Obstetrics & Gynecology, 133(3), 323-352.* https://doi.org/10.1016/0002-9378(79)90688-4

Gottfreðsdottir, H., Small, K., Helgadottir, B., & Gamble, J. (2025). Who is in the centre? A qualitative study on midwives' experience of working with central fetal monitoring system. *Women & Birth, 38(2), 101891.* https://doi.org/10.1016/j.wombi.2025.101891

Grant, A., Joy, M.-T., O'Brien, N., Hennessy, E., & MacDonald, D. (1989). Cerebral palsy among children born during the Dublin trial randomised trial of intrapartum monitoring. *Lancet, 334(8674), 1233-1236.* https://www.ncbi.nlm.nih.gov/pubmed/2573757

Grivell, R. M., Alfirevic, Z., Gyte, G. M., & Devane, D. (2015). Antenatal cardiotocography for fetal assessment. *Cochrane Database of Systematic Reviews, 2015(9), CD007863.* https://doi.org/10.1002/14651858.CD007863.pub4

Grobman, W., Rice, M., Reddy, U., Tita, A., Silver, R., Mallett, G., Hill, K., ... & Eunice Kennedy Shriver National Institute of Child Health and Human Development Maternal-Fetal Medicine Units Network. (2018). Labor induction versus expectant management in low-risk nulliparous women. *New England Journal of Medicine, 379(6), 513-523.* https://doi.org/10.1056/NEJMoa1800566

Habraken, V., Spanjers, M., van der Woude, D., Oei, S., & van Laar, J. (2022). Experiences with intrapartum fetal monitoring in the Netherlands: A survey study. *European Journal of Obstetrics & Gynecology & Reproductive Biology, 278, 159-165.* https://www.ncbi.nlm.nih.gov/pubmed/36208521

Hammad, I. A., Chauhan, S., Magann, E., & Abuhamad, A. (2013). Peripartum complications with cesarean delivery: a review of Maternal-Fetal Medicine Units Network publications. *The Journal of Maternal-Fetal & Neonatal Medicine, 27(5), 463-474.* http://www.tandfonline.com/doi/full/10.3109/14767058.2013.818970

Hancox, R., Landhuis, C., & Sears, M. (2013). Forceps birth delivery, allergic sensitisation and asthma: a population-based cohort study. *Clinical & Experimental Allergy, 43(3), 332-336.* https://www.ncbi.nlm.nih.gov/pubmed/23414541

Harper, L., Shanks, A., Tuuli, M., Roehl, K., & Cahill, A. (2013). The risks and benefits of internal monitors in laboring patients. *American Journal of Obstetrics & Gynecology, 209(1), 38.e31-36.* http://linkinghub.elsevier.com/retrieve/pii/S0002937813003505

Hautakangas, T., Uotila, J., Huhtala, H., & Palomaki, O. (2020). Intrauterine versus external tocodynamometry in monitoring labour: a randomised controlled clinical trial. *British Journal of Obstetrics & Gynaecology, 127(13), 1677-1686.* https://www.ncbi.nlm.nih.gov/pubmed/32491233

Haverkamp, A., Thompson, H., McFee, J., & Cetrulo, C. (1976). The evaluation of continuous fetal heart rate monitoring in high-risk pregnancy. *American Journal of Obstetrics & Gynecology, 125(3), 310-320.* https://www.ncbi.nlm.nih.gov/pubmed/5895

Haverkamp, A., Orleans, M., Langendoerfer, S., McFee, J., Murphy, J., & Thompson, H. (1979). A controlled trial of the differential effects of intrapartum fetal monitoring. *American Journal of Obstetrics & Gynecology, 134(4), 399-412.* https://www.ncbi.nlm.nih.gov/pubmed/453276

Hayes-Gill, B., Martin, T., Liu, C., & Cohen, W. (2020). Relative accuracy of computerized intrapartum fetal heart rate pattern recognition by ultrasound and abdominal electrocardiogram detection. *Acta Obstetrica et Gynecologica Scandinavica, 99(3), 413-422.* https://www.ncbi.nlm.nih.gov/pubmed/31792930

Health Service Executive National Women and Infants Programme. (2021). *National Clinical Guideline for Intrapartum Fetal Heart Rate Monitoring.* https://irelandsouthwid.cumh.hse.ie/maternity/labour-delivery/stages-of-labour/national-clinical-guideline-for-intrapartum-fetal-heart-rate-monitoring-2021-.pdf

Heelan-Fancher, L., Shi, L., Zhang, Y., Cai, Y., Nawai, A., & Leveille, S. (2019). Impact of continuous electronic fetal monitoring on birth outcomes in low-risk pregnancies. *Birth, 46(2), 311-317.* https://www.ncbi.nlm.nih.gov/pubmed/30811649

Herbst, A., & Ingemarsson, I. (1994). Intermittent versus continuous electronic monitoring in labour: a randomised study. *British Journal of Obstetrics & Gynaecology, 101(8), 663-668.* https://doi.org/10.1111/j.1471-0528.1994.tb13181.x

Hindley, C., Hinsliff, S., & Thomson, A. (2006). English midwives' views and experiences of intrapartum fetal heart rate monitoring in women at low obstetric risk: conflicts and compromises. *Journal of Midwifery & Women's Health, 51(5), 354–360.* https://www.ncbi.nlm.nih.gov/pubmed/16945783

Hindley, C., Hinsliff, S., & Thomson, A. (2008). Pregnant womens' views about choice of intrapartum monitoring of the fetal heart rate: A questionnaire survey. *International Journal of Nursing Studies, 45(2), 224-231.* https://doi.org/10.1016/j.ijnurstu.2006.08.019

Hindley, C., & Thomson, A. (2005). The rhetoric of informed choice: perspectives from midwives on intrapartum fetal heart rate monitoring. *Health Expectations, 8(4), 306-314.* https://doi.org/10.1111/j.1369-7625.2005.00355.x

Hollowell, J., Puddicombe, D., Rowe, R., Linsell, L., Hardy, P., Stewart, M., Redshaw, M., ... & Birthplace in England Collaborative Group. (2011). *The Birthplace national prospective cohort study: perinatal and maternal outcomes by planned place of birth Birthplace in England research programme.* http://openaccess.city. ac.uk/3650/1/Birthplace_Clinical_Report_SDO_FR4_08-1604-140_V03.pdf

Homer, C., Cheah, S., Rossiter, C., Dahlen, H., Ellwood, D., Foureur, M., Forster, D., ... & Scarf, V. (2019). Maternal and perinatal outcomes by planned place of birth in Australia 2000 - 2012: a linked population data study. *BMJ Open, 9(10), e029192.* https://www.ncbi.nlm.nih.gov/pubmed/31662359

Hon, E. (1958). The electronic evaluation of the fetal heart rate; preliminary report. *American Journal of Obstetrics & Gynecology, 75(6), 1215-1230.* https:// doi.org/10.1016/0002-9378(58)90707-5

Hsieh, W-S., Yang, P-H., Chao, H-C., & Lai, J-Y. (1999). Neonatal necrotizing fasciitis: A report of three cases and review of the literature. *Pediatrics, 103(4),e53.* https://doi.org/10.1542/peds.103.4.e53

INFANT Collaborative Group. (2017). Computerised interpretation of fetal heart rate during labour (INFANT): a randomised controlled trial. *The Lancet, 389(10080), 1719-1729.* https://www.ncbi.nlm.nih.gov/pubmed/28341515

Jepsen, I., Blix, E., Cooke, H., Adrian, S. W., & Maude, R. (2022). The overuse of intrapartum cardiotocography (CTG) for low-risk women: An actor-network theory analysis of data from focus groups. *Women & Birth, 35(6), 593-601.* https://doi.org/10.1016/j.wombi.2022.01.003

Johnson, G. J., Salmanian, B., Denning, S. G., Belfort, M. A., Sundgren, N. C., & Clark, S. L. (2021). Relationship between umbilical cord gas values and neonatal outcomes: Implications for electronic fetal heart rate monitoring. *Obstetrics & Gynecology, 138(3), 366-373. https://doi.org/10.1097/AOG.0000000000004515*

Kalter, H. (1991). Five-decade international trends in the relation of perinatal mortality and congenital malformations: Stillbirth and neonatal death compared. International Journal of Epidemiology, 20(1), 173-179. https://www. ncbi.nlm.nih.gov/pubmed/1712348

Kang, J., Koehler, R., Graham, E., & Boctor, E. (2021). Photoacoustic assessment of the fetal brain and placenta as a method of non-invasive antepartum and intrapartum monitoring. *Experimental Neurology, 347, 113898.* https://www. ncbi.nlm.nih.gov/pubmed/34662542

Kasap, B., Vali, K., Qian, W., Mo, L., Chithiwala, Z., Curtin, A., Ghiasi, S., & Hedriana, H. (2024). Transcutaneous discrimination of fetal heart rate from maternal heart rate: A fetal oximetry proof-of-concept. *Reproductive Sciences, 31(8), 2331-2341.* https://doi.org/10.1007/s43032-024-01582-z

Kawakita, T., Reddy, U., Landy, H., Iqbal, S., Huang, C.-C., & Grantz, K. (2016). Neonatal complications associated with use of fetal scalp electrode: a retrospective study. *British Journal of Obstetrics & Gynaecology, 123(11), 1797-1803.* https://www.ncbi.nlm.nih.gov/pubmed/26643181

Keag, O., Norman, J., & Stock, S. (2018). Long-term risks and benefits associated with cesarean delivery for mother, baby, and subsequent pregnancies: Systematic review and meta-analysis. *PLoS Medicine, 15(1), e1002494-1002422.* http://dx.plos.org/10.1371/journal.pmed.1002494

Kearney, R., Fitzpatrick, M., Brennan, S., Behan, M., Miller, J., Keane, D., O'Herlihy, C., & DeLancey, J. (2010). Levator ani injury in primiparous women with forceps delivery for fetal distress, forceps for second stage arrest, and spontaneous delivery. *International Journal of Gynecology & Obstetrics, 111(1), 19-22.* https://www.ncbi.nlm.nih.gov/pubmed/20650455

Kelso, I., Parsons, R., Lawrence, G., Arora, S., Edmonds, D., & Cooke, I. (1978). An assessment of continuous fetal heart rate monitoring in labor. A randomized trial. *American Journal of Obstetrics & Gynecology, 131(5), 526-532.* https://www.ncbi.nlm.nih.gov/pubmed/677195

Knupp, R., Andrews, W., & Tita, A. (2020). The future of electronic fetal monitoring. *Best Practice & Research in Clinical Obstetrics & Gynaecology, 67, 44-52.* https://www.ncbi.nlm.nih.gov/pubmed/32269728

Kuah, S., Simpson, B., Salter, A., Matthews, G., Louise, J., Bednarz, J., Chandraharan, E., Symonds, I., McPhee, A., Mol, B., Turnbull, D., & Wilkinson, C. (2023). Comparison of effect of CTG + STan with CTG alone on emergency cesarean section rate: STan Australian Randomized controlled Trial (START). *Ultrasound in Obstetrics & Gynecology, 62(4), 462-470.* https://doi.org/10.1002/uog.26279

Lear, C., Galinsky, R., Wassink, G., Yamaguchi, K., Davidson, J., Westgate, J., Bennet, L., & Gunn, A. (2016). The myths and physiology surrounding intrapartum decelerations: the critical role of the peripheral chemoreflex. *Journal of Physiology, 594(17), 4711-4725.* http://doi.wiley.com/10.1113/JP271205

Lear, C., Wassink, G., Westgate, J., Nijhuis, J., Ugwumadu, A., Galinsky, R., Bennet, L., & Gunn, A. (2018). The peripheral chemoreflex: indefatigable guardian of fetal physiological adaptation to labour. *Journal of Physiology, 596(23), 5611-5623*. https://www.ncbi.nlm.nih.gov/pubmed/29604081

Lear, C., Westgate, J., Bennet, L., Ugwumadu, A., Stone, P., Tournier, A., & Gunn, A. (2023). Fetal defenses against intrapartum head compression – implications for intrapartum decelerations and hypoxic-ischemic injury. *American Journal of Obstetrics & Gynecololgy, 228(5S), S1117-S1128*. https://doi.org/10.1016/j.ajog.2021.11.1352

Lee, S., & Hon, E. (1963). Fetal hemodynamic response to umbilical cord compression. *Obstetrics & Gynecology, 22, 553–562*. https://www.ncbi.nlm.nih.gov/pubmed/14082272

Leveno, K., Cunningham, F., Nelson, S., Roark, M., Williams, M., Guzick, D., Dowling, S., Rosenfeld, C., & Buckley, A. (1986). A prospective comparison of selective and universal electronic fetal monitoring in 34,995 pregnancies. *New England Journal of Medicine, 315(10), 615-619*. https://www.ncbi.nlm.nih.gov/pubmed/3736600

Levett, K., Fox, D., Bamhare, P., Sutcliffe, K., Coddington, R., Newnham, L., & Scarf, V. (2024). Do women have a choice when it comes to fetal monitoring? Perceptions of information provided and choice of fetal monitoring in Australia: A national survey. *Women & Birth, 37(6), 101837*. https://doi.org/10.1016/j.wombi.2024.101837

Levett, K., Sutcliffe, K., Vanderlaan, J., & Kjerulff, K. (2024). The First Baby Study: What women would like to have known about first childbirth. A mixed-methods study. *Birth, 51(4), 795-805*. https://doi.org/10.1111/birt.12854

Liljeström, L., Wikström, A.-K., Skalkidou, A., Åkerud, H., & Jonsson, M. (2014). Experience of fetal scalp blood sampling during labor. *Acta Obstetricia et Gynecologica Scandinavica, 93(1), 113-117*. https://www.ncbi.nlm.nih.gov/pubmed/24116986

Lindquist, S., Shah, N., Overgaard, C., Torp-Pedersen, C., Glavind, K., Larsen, T., Plough, A., Galvin, G., & Knudsen, A. (2017). Association of previous cesarean delivery with surgical complications after a hysterectomy later in life. *JAMA Surgery, 152(12), 1148-1155*. https://www.ncbi.nlm.nih.gov/pubmed/28793157

Liston, R. M., Sawchuck, D., & Young, D. (2018). No. 197b - Fetal health surveillance: Intrapartum consensus guideline. *Journal of Obstetrics & Gynaecology Canada, 40(4), e298-e322.* https://doi.org/10.1016/j.jogc.2018.02.011

Logan, R., McLemore, M., Julian, Z., Stoll, K., Malhotra, N., GVtM Steering Council, & Vedam, S. (2022). Coercion and non-consent during birth and newborn care in the United States. *Birth, 49(4), 749-762.* https://doi.org/10.1111/birt.12641

Luthy, D., Shy, K., van Belle, G., Larson, E., Hughes, J., Benedetti, T., Brown, Z., Effer, S., King, J., & Stenchever, M. (1987). A randomized trial of electronic fetal monitoring in preterm labor. *Obstetrics & Gynecology, 69(5), 687-695.* https://www.ncbi.nlm.nih.gov/pubmed/3554055

MacDonald, D., Grant, A., Sheridan-Pereira, M., Boylan, P., & Chalmers, I. (1985). The Dublin randomized controlled trial of intrapartum fetal heart rate monitoring. *American Journal of Obstetrics & Gynecology, 152(5), 524-539.* https://www.ncbi.nlm.nih.gov/pubmed/3893132

Madaan, M., & Trivedi, S. (2006). Intrapartum electronic fetal monitoring vs. intermittent auscultation in postcesarean pregnancies. *International Journal of Gynecology & Obstetrics, 94(2), 123-125.* http://doi.wiley.com/10.1016/j.ijgo.2006.03.026

Mancuso, A., De Vivo, A., Fanara, G., Denaro, A., Laganà, D., & Maria Accardo, F. (2008). Effects of antepartum electronic fetal monitoring on maternal emotional state. *Acta Obstetricia et Gynecologica Scandinavica, 87(2), 184-189.* http://doi.wiley.com/10.1080/00016340701823892

Mascarello, K., Horta, B., & Silveira, M. (2017). Maternal complications and cesarean section without indication: systematic review and meta-analysis. *Revista de Saude Publica, 51, 105.* https://www.ncbi.nlm.nih.gov/pubmed/29166440

McAnena, L., O'Keefe, M., Kirwan, C., & Murphy, J. (2015). Forceps delivery-related ophthalmic injuries: A case series. *Journal of Pediatric Ophthalmology and Strabismus, 52(6), 355-359.* https://www.ncbi.nlm.nih.gov/pubmed/26584749

McDonald, E., Gartland, D., Small, R., & Brown, S. (2015). Dyspareunia and childbirth: a prospective cohort study. *British Journal of Obstetrics and Gynaecology, 122, 672-679.* http://onlinelibrary.wiley.com/doi/10.1111/1471-0528.13263/full

McMahon, G., Rogers, A., Woulfe, Z., Tuthill, E., Doyle, M., Burke, G., & Imcha, M. (2019). Women's opinions on cardiotocograph monitoring and staff communication during labour. *Irish Medical Journal, 112(10), 1022.* https://www.ncbi.nlm.nih.gov/pubmed/32311252

Miller, Y., Tone, J., Talukdar, S., & Martin, E. (2022). A direct comparison of patient-reported outcomes and experiences in alternative models of maternity care in Queensland, Australia. *PLoS ONE, 17(7), e0271105.* https://doi.org/10.1371/journal.pone.0271105

Mires, S., Kerr, R. S., Denbow, M., Dahnoun, N., Tancock, S., Osredkar, D., & Chakkarapani, E. (2022). Foetal amplitude-integrated electroencephalography: proof of principle of a novel foetal monitoring technique in adult volunteers. *Journal of Obstetrics & Gynaecology, 42(7), 2672-2679.* https://doi.org/10.1080/01443615.2022.2081797

Morris, Z., Wooding, S., & Grant, J. (2011). The answer is 17 years, what is the question: understanding time lags in translational research. *Journal of the Royal Society of Medicine, 104(12), 510-520. doi:*10.1258/jrsm.2011.110180

Munro, J., Ford, H., Scott, A., Furnival, E., Andrews, S., & Grayson, A. (2002). Action research project responding to midwives' views of different methods of fetal monitoring in labour. *MIDIRS: Midwifery Digest, 12(4), 495–498.*

National Institute for Health and Care Excellence. (2022). Fetal monitoring in labour. www.nice.org.uk/guidance/ng229

Newnham, E., & Kirkham, M. (2019). Beyond autonomy: Care ethics for midwifery and the humanization of birth. *Nursing Ethics, 26(7-8), 096973301881911.* https://doi.org/10.1177/0969733018819119

Newnham, E. C., McKellar, L. V., & Pincombe, J. I. (2017). "It's your body, but..." Mixed messages in childbirth education: Findings from a hospital ethnography. *Midwifery, 55, 53-59.* https://doi.org/10.1016/j.midw.2017.09.003

Nordström, L., Achanna, S., Naka, K., & Arulkumaran, S. (2001). Fetal and maternal lactate increase during active second stage of labour. *British Journal of Obstetrics & Gynaecology, 108(3), 263-268.* https://doi.org/10.1016/S0306-5456(00)00034-6

Nunes, I., Ayres-de-Campos, D., Ugwumadu, A., Amin, P., Banfield, P., Nicoll, A., Cunningham, S., Sousa, P., Costa-Santos, C., & Bernardes, J. (2017). Central fetal monitoring with and without computer analysis. A randomized controlled trial. *Obstetrics & Gynecology, 129(1), 83-90*. https://doi.org/10.1097/AOG.0000000000001799

Ockenden, D. (2022). *Findings, conclusions and essential actions from the independent review of maternity services at the Shrewsbury and Telford Hospital NHS Trust*. www.gov.uk/official-documents

Oláh, K. S., & Steer, P. J. (2015). The use and abuse of oxytocin. *The Obstetrician & Gynaecologist, 17(4), 265-271*. https://doi.org/10.1111/tog.12222

Olofsson, P. (2023). Umbilical cord pH, blood gases, and lactate at birth: normal values, interpretation, and clinical utility. *American Journal of Obstetrics & Gynecology, 228(5S), S1222-S1240*. https://doi.org/10.1016/j.ajog.2022.07.001

Peters, L., Thornton, C., de Jonge, A., Khashan, A., Tracy, M., Downe, S., Feijen-de Jong, E., & Dahlen, H. (2018). The effect of medical and operative birth interventions on child health outcomes in the first 28 days and up to 5 years of age: A linked data population-based cohort study. *Birth, 11, 347-357*. http://doi.wiley.com/10.1111/birt.12348

Phillips. (2007). Fetal spiral electrode. Instructions for use. https://www.documents.philips.com/assets/Instruction%20for%20Use/20231108/2a3e806753af4fd797cab0b40132507b.pdf

Pinkerton, J. H. (1969). Kergaradec, friend of Laennec and pioneer of foetal auscultation. *Proceeds of the Royal Society of Medicine, 62(5), 477-483*. https://www.ncbi.nlm.nih.gov/pubmed/4890358

Polidano, C., Zhu, A., & Bornstein, J. (2017). The relation between cesarean birth and child cognitive development. *Scientific Reports, 7(1), 11483*. http://www.nature.com/articles/s41598-017-10831-y

Rabe, H., Gyte, G., Díaz-Rossello, J., & Duley, L. (2019). Effect of timing of umbilical cord clamping and other strategies to influence placental transfusion at preterm birth on maternal and infant outcomes. *Cochrane Database of Systematic Reviews, 9, CD003248*. https://doi.org/10.1002/14651858.CD003248.pub4

Reavis, L. (2011). *Effect of Remote Fetal Monitoring in an Inpatient Obstetrical Unit: A Retrospective Review. Masters thesis. Gardner-Webb University. Boiling Springs.* https://digitalcommons.gardner-webb.edu/nursing_etd/166/

Renou, P., Chang, A., Anderson, I., & Wood, C. (1976). Controlled trial of fetal intensive care. *American Journal of Obstetrics & Gynecology, 126(4), 470-476.* https://www.ncbi.nlm.nih.gov/pubmed/10731

Reynolds, A., Murray, M., Geary, M., Ater, S., & Hayes, B. (2022). Fetal heart rate patterns in labor and the risk of neonatal encephalopathy: A case control study. *European Journal of Obstetrics & Gynecology & Reproductive Biology, 273, 69-74.* https://www.ncbi.nlm.nih.gov/pubmed/35504116

Roebuck, C., Sandall, J., West, R., *Atherden, A., Parkyn, K., & Johnson, O. (2025). Impact of midwife continuity of carer on stillbirth rate and first feed in England. Commununications Medicine, 5, 339 (2025).* https://doi.org/10.1038/s43856-025-01025-z

Rodgers, C. (2020). Continuous electronic fetal monitoring during prolonged labor may be a risk factor for having a child diagnosed with autism spectrum disorder. *Medical Hypotheses, 145, 110339.* https://www.ncbi.nlm.nih.gov/pubmed/33126162

Rodgers, C. (2025). Why do more boys than girls develop autism? ResearchGate preprint. https://www.researchgate.net/publication/392027363_RodgersWhy_do_more_boys_than_girls_develop_autismPREPRINT_revised_5-23-25?_=eyJj b250ZXh0Ijp7InBhZ2UiOiJtZXNzYWdlcyIsInByZXZpb3VzUGFnZSI6bnVsbH19

Rood, K. (2012). Complications associated with insertion of intrauterine pressure catheters: an unusual case of uterine hypertonicity and uterine perforation resulting in fetal distress after insertion of an intrauterine pressure catheter. *Case Reports in Obstetrics & Gynecology, 2012, 517461.* https://www.ncbi.nlm.nih.gov/pubmed/22928133

Rosén, K. G., Hökegård, K. H., & Kjellmer, I. (1976). A study of the relationship between the electrocardiogram and hemodynamics in the fetal lamb during asphyxia. *Acta Physiologica Scandinavica, 98(3), 275-284.* https://doi.org/10.1111/j.1748-1716.1976.tb10312.x

Royal Australian and New Zealand College of Obstetricians and Gynaecologists. (2019). *Intrapartum fetal surveillance clinical guideline. 4th Edn. (Now replaced.)*

Royal Australian and New Zealand College of Obstetricians and Gynaecologists. (2025). *Intrapartum fetal surveillance clinical guideline. 5th Edn.* https://ranzcog.edu.au/statements-guidelines

Sadowska, M., Sarecka-Hujar, B., & Kopyta, I. (2020). Cerebral palsy: Current opinions on definition, epidemiology, risk factors, classification and treatment options. *Neuropsychiatric Disease & Treatment, 16, 1505-1518.* https://doi.org/10.2147/NDT.S235165

Sandall, J., Fernandez Turienzo, C., Devane, D., Soltani, H., Gillespie, P., Gates, S., Jones, L., Shennan, A., & Rayment-Jones, H. (2024). Midwife continuity of care models versus other models of care for childbearing women. *Cochrane Database of Systematic Reviews, 4(4), CD004667.* https://doi.org/10.1002/14651858.CD004667.pub6

Schroeder, E., Yang, M., Brocklehurst, P., Linsell, L., & Rivero-Arias, O. (2020). Economic evaluation of computerised interpretation of fetal heart rate during labour: a cost-consequence analysis alongside the INFANT study. *Archives of Diseases in Childhood. Fetal & Neonatal Edition, 106(2), 143-148.* https://www.ncbi.nlm.nih.gov/pubmed/32796054

Sevelsted, A., Stokholm, J., Bønnelykke, K., & Bisgaard, H. (2015). Cesarean section and chronic immune disorders. *Pediatrics, 135(1), e92-98.* https://www.ncbi.nlm.nih.gov/pubmed/25452656

Shalev, E., Eran, A., Harpaz-kerpel, S., & Zuckerman, H. (1985). Psychogenic stress in women during fetal monitoring (hormonal profile). *Acta Obstetricia et Gynecologica Scandinavica, 64(5), 417-420.* https://www.ncbi.nlm.nih.gov/pubmed/3904314

Shy, K., Luthy, D., Bennett, F., Whitfield, M., Larson, E., van Belle, G., Hughes, J., Wilson, J., & Stenchever, M. (1990). Effects of electronic fetal-heart-rate monitoring, as compared with periodic auscultation, on the neurologic development of premature infants. *New England Journal of Medicine, 322(9), 588-593.* https://www.ncbi.nlm.nih.gov/pubmed/3554055

Siddiqi, S., & Taylor, P. (1982). Necrotizing fasciitis of the scalp: a complication of fetal monitoring. *American Journal of Diseases of Children, 136, 226-228.* https://www.ncbi.nlm.nih.gov/pubmed/7064948

Slabuszewska-Jozwiak, A., Szymanski, J., Ciebiera, M., Sarecka-Hujar, B., & Jakiel, G. (2020). Pediatrics consequences of caesarean section - A systematic review and meta-analysis. *International Journal of Environmental Research & Public Health, 17(21).* https://www.ncbi.nlm.nih.gov/pubmed/33142727

Small, K. (2025). Whose CTG data is it? https://birthsmalltalk.com/2025/04/02/whose-ctg-data-is-it/

Small, K., Sidebotham, M., Fenwick, J., & Gamble, J. (2020). Intrapartum cardiotocograph monitoring and perinatal outcomes for women at risk: Literature review. *Women & Birth, 33(5), 411-418.* https://www.ncbi.nlm.nih.gov/pubmed/31668871

Small, K., Sidebotham, M., Fenwick, J., & Gamble, J. (2022). "I'm not doing what I should be doing as a midwife": An ethnographic exploration of central fetal monitoring and perceptions of clinical safety. *Women & Birth, 35(2), 193-200.* https://www.ncbi.nlm.nih.gov/pubmed/34092530

Small, K., Sidebotham, M., Fenwick, J., & Gamble, J. (2023). The social organisation of decision-making about intrapartum fetal monitoring: An Institutional Ethnography. *Women & Birth, 36(3), 281-289.* https://doi.org/10.1016/j.wombi.2022.09.004

Smith, G., & Pell, J. (2003). Parachute use to prevent death and major trauma related to gravitational challenge: systematic review of randomised controlled trials. *British Medical Journal, 327(7429), 1459-1461.* https://www.ncbi.nlm.nih.gov/pubmed/14684649

Smith, V., Begley, C., & Devane, D. (2017). Technology in childbirth: Exploring women's views of fetal monitoring during labour - a systematic review. In S. Church, L. Frith, M. Balsam, M. Berg, V. Smith, C. van der Walt, S. Downe, & E. van Teijlingen (Eds.), *New thinking on improving maternity care: International perspectives (pp. 170-193). Pinter and Martin.*

Smith, V., Begley, C., Newell, J., Higgins, S., Murphy, D., White, M., Morrison, J., ... & Devane, D. (2018). Admission cardiotocography versus intermittent auscultation of the fetal heart in low-risk pregnancy during evaluation for possible labour admission - a multicentre randomised trial: The ADCAR trial. *British Journal of Obstetrics & Gynaecology, 126(1), 114-121.* https://dx.doi. org/10.1111/1471-0528.15448=

Sterne, J., Hernan, M., Reeves, B., Savovic, J., Berkman, N., Viswanathan, M., Henry, D., et al. (2016). ROBINS-I: a tool for assessing risk of bias in non-randomised studies of interventions. *British Medical Journak, 355, i4919.* https://doi.org/10.1136/bmj.i4919

Stone, P., Burgess, W., McIntyre, J., Gunn, A., Lear, C., Bennet, L., Mitchell, E., Thompson, J., & the Maternal Sleep in Pregnancy Research Group. (2017). Effect of maternal position on fetal behavioural state and heart rate variability in healthy late gestation pregnancy. *Journal of Physiology, 595(4), 1213-1221.* https://www.ncbi.nlm.nih.gov/pubmed/27871127

Tahmina, S., Daniel, M., & Krishnan, L. (2022). Manual fetal stimulation during intrapartum fetal surveillance: a randomized controlled trial. *American Journal of Obstetrics & Gynecology Maternal Fetal Medicine, 4(2), 100574.* https://www. ncbi.nlm.nih.gov/pubmed/35051669

Talmor, M., Rotem, R., Wientraub, A., & Yaniv Salem, S. (2023). The correlation between total deceleration and acceleration surface areas on electronic fetal monitoring and neonatal cord blood pH in postdate pregnancies. *International Journal of Gynaecology & Obstetrics, 161(3), 870-876.* https://doi.org/10.1002/ ijgo.14558

Taylor, B., Cross-Sudworth, F., Rimmer, M. Quinn, L., Morris, R. K., Johnston, T., Morad, S., Davidson, L., Kenyon, S., UK Audit & Research Collaborative in Obstetrics & Gynaecology Members. (2024). Induction of labour care in the UK: A cross-sectional survey of maternity units. *PLoS ONE, 19(2), e0297857.* https:// doi.org/10.1371/journal.pone.0297857

Thompson, M. S. (1981). Decision-analytic determination of study size. The case of electronic fetal monitoring. *Medical Decision Making, 1(2), 165-179.* https:// www.ncbi.nlm.nih.gov/pubmed/6763124

Thompson, R., & Miller, Y. (2014). Birth control: To what extent do women report being informed and involved in decisions about pregnancy and birth procedures? *BMC Pregnancy and Childbirth, 14, 62.* http://www.biomedcentral. com/1471-2393/14/62

Tournier, A., Beacom, M., Westgate, J., Bennet, L., Garabedian, C., Ugwumadu, A., Gunn, A., & Lear, C. (2021). Physiological control of fetal heart rate variability during labour: Implications and controversies. *Journal of Physiology, 600(3), 431-450.* https://www.ncbi.nlm.nih.gov/pubmed/34951476

Tsipoura, A., Giaxi, P., Sarantaki, A., & Gourounti, K. (2023). Conventional cardiotocography versus computerized CTG analysis and perinatal outcomes: A systematic review. *Maedica: A Journal of Clinical Medicine, 18(3), 483-489.* https://doi.org/10.26574/maedica.2023.18.3.483

Valenzuela, C., Gregory, E., & Martin, J. (2023). *Perinatal mortality in the United States, 2020-2021. NCHS data brief, no 489. Hyattsville, MD: National Center for Health Statistics. DOI:* https://dx.doi.org/10.15620/cdc:134756

Vintzileos, A., Antsaklis, A., Varvarigos, I., Papas, C., Sofatzis, I., & Montgomery, J. (1993). A randomized trial of intrapartum electronic fetal heart rate monitoring versus intermittent auscultation. *Obstetrics & Gynecology, 81(6), 899-907.* https://www.ncbi.nlm.nih.gov/pubmed/8497353

Volløyhaug, I., Mørkved, S., Salvesen, Ø., & Salvesen, K. (2015). Forceps delivery is associated with increased risk of pelvic organ prolapse and muscle trauma: a cross-sectional study 16-24 years after first delivery. *Ultrasound in Obstetrics & Gynecology, 46(4), 487-495.* https://www.ncbi.nlm.nih.gov/pubmed/25920322

Walker, D., Shunkwiler, S., Supanich, J., Williamsen, J., & Yensch, A. (2001). Labor and delivery nurse's attitudes towards intermittent fetal monitoring. *Journal of Midwifery & Women's Health, 46(6), 374-380.* https://www.ncbi.nlm.nih.gov/pubmed/11783685

Walker, N. (1959). The case for conservatism in management of foetal distress. *British Journal of Medicine, 2(5161), 1221-1226.* https://www.ncbi.nlm.nih.gov/pubmed/13842533

Watson, K., Mills, T., & Lavender, T. (2022). Experiences and outcomes on the use of telemetry to monitor the fetal heart during labour: findings from a mixed methods study. *Women & Birth, 35(3), e243-e252.* https://doi.org/10.1016/j.wombi.2021.06.004

Weiss, P., Balducci, J., Reed, J., Klasko, S., & Rust, O. (1997). Does centralized monitoring affect perinatal outcome? *Journal of Maternal-Fetal & Neonatal Medicine, 6(6), 317-319.* http://www.tandfonline.com/doi/full/10.3109/14767059709162013

Wendland, C. (2007). The vanishing mother: Cesarean section and "evidence-based obstetrics". *Medical Anthropology Quarterly, 21(2), 218-233.* https://www.ncbi.nlm.nih.gov/pubmed/17601085

Wiberg-Itzel, E., Wray, S., & Åkerud, H. (2018). A randomized controlled trial of a new treatment for labor dystocia. *Journal of Maternal-Fetal & Neonatal Medicine, 31(17), 2237-2244.* https://doi.org/10.1080/14767058.2017.1339268

Withiam-Leitch, M., Shelton, J., & Fleming, E. (2006). Central fetal monitoring: effect on perinatal outcomes and cesarean section rate. *Birth, 33(4), 284-288.* http://doi.wiley.com/10.1111/j.1523-536X.2006 00120.x

Wood, C., Renou, P., Oats, J., Farrell, E.-M., Beischer, N., & Anderson, I. (1981). A controlled trial of fetal heart rate monitoring in a low-risk obstetric population. *American Journal of Obstetrics & Gynecology, 141(5), 527-534.* https://www.ncbi.nlm.nih.gov/pubmed/7294080

Yambasu, S., Boland, F., O'Donoghue, K., Curran, C., Shahabuddin, Y., Cotter, A., Gaffney, G., Devane, D., Molloy, E. J., & Murphy, D. J. (2025). Digital foetal scalp stimulation versus foetal blood sampling to assess foetal well-being in labour: A multicentre randomised controlled trial. *BJOG, 132(5), 557-564.* https://doi.org/10.1111/1471-0528.18068

Acknowledgements

No work of this nature is possible without the support of a great many people, and not all of them appear in this acknowledgement.

To Tara and Ryan, my grown up babies. Your love and support lifts me up. Baby Harvey (born while this book was gestating) begins the next generation of our family.

My PhD supervisors Professors Jennifer Fenwick, Jenny Gamble, and Mary Sidebotham were instrumental in the development of my knowledge, research ability, and writing skills. While not involved directly in the creation of this book, without their earlier guidance and support it would not have been possible for me to dream it up and make it happen.

A huge thank you to the thousands and thousands of people who have read, commented on, and shared my blog posts. Knowing that my work makes a material difference in people's lives inspires me to keep at it. I also want to acknowledge the many dedicated researchers who have published, and continue to produce fetal monitoring research. That research helps maternity professionals, and the people who use their services, to make informed decisions and constantly strive to achieve maternity care systems that work effectively for all.

Thanks go to Dr Sara Wickham, the original birth blogger, influencer, and author. You carved out a path for others, including myself, to follow. Your advice and support over the years has been greatly appreciated. And to Dr Melanie Jackson, whose bright entrepreneurial spirit reminds me to just do the thing and stop trying to get it "perfect"!

Dr Nadine Edwards provided professional editing services during the creation of the book. Her generous feedback helped make the book better than I could have managed on my own. Deb Parker from Mookoo Designs made the wonderful illustrations and cover art that help to bring my words to life. Sophie White for typesetting the book so beautifully. Julie Postance, Elizabeth Lyons, and Catherine Deveny taught me how to publish and Leonie Dawson taught me how to promote and sell the book.

To Professor Susan Bewley and Catherine Williams, who along with Dr Carolyn Hastie and the members of the Friday morning writing group helped to keep me turning up at the writing desk – thank you for your gentle encouragement.

About the author

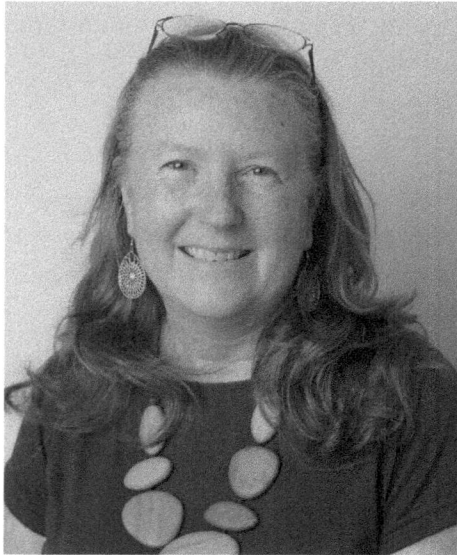

Dr Kirsten Small BMedSc, MBBS, MReproMed, GradDipHlthRes, PhD

Dr Kirsten Small is a retired specialist obstetrician and gynaecologist. She works as an educator, researcher, and writer. For many years, Kirsten has shared her detailed knowledge about fetal monitoring through her informative and accessible blog Birth Small Talk. She is motivated by the vision of promoting and protecting respectful maternity care for women, babies, families, and their care providers. As a feminist, Kirsten is critical of patriarchal values embedded in maternity care systems, and particularly within obstetrics and gynaecology.

Kirsten lives on Gubbi Gubbi land on the Sunshine Coast, Queensland, Australia. She is mother to two lovely grown up people and now a grandmother.

Looking for more information?

The Birth Small Talk blog will help you learn more about the evidence about every aspect of fetal heart rate monitoring. Subscribe to be notified whenever a new blog post is published.

birthsmalltalk.com

I offer online education for maternity professionals, other birth workers, and women planning their birth. For more information, subscribe to the monthly Birth Small Talk newsletter.

education.birthsmalltalk.com/newsletter

www.ingramcontent.com/pod-product-compliance
Lightning Source LLC
Chambersburg PA
CBHW051245020426
42333CB00025B/3060